FASTING for METABOLISM

The Quick & Easy Way To Brunch Yourself Thin

Kate Hardy

Copyright © 2025 by Kate Hardy

All rights reserved.

No part of this book may be reproduced in any form or by any electronic or mechanical means, including information storage and retrieval systems, without written permission from the author, except for the use of brief quotations in a book review.

Contents

1. Does Your Metabolism Need a Reset? — 1
2. How Life Sabotages Diet — 8
3. Timing - The Secret Ingredient for a Faster Metabolism — 13
4. Making Intermittent Fasting Work for You — 17
5. Building The Perfect Brunch — 22
6. A Light & Later Lunch… Replaces Snacking — 38
7. The Golden Rules of Evening — 41
8. Cheat Days — 48
9. Bonus Diet Hack — 51
10. The Right Exercise Can Supercharge Your Results — 55
11. Timing Your Workout — 70
12. Real Life Routines — 73
13. 5 Habits That Change Everything — 77
14. Metabolism & Menopause — 80
15. Mindset & Motivation — 85
16. The Habit Challenge — 92
17. A New Blueprint for Modern Women — 95

Appendices

Appendix 1: A Sample 7-Day Meal Plan — 101
Appendix 2: Macros Reference Table — 110
Appendix 3: FAQs About Intermittent Fasting, Meal Timing, and Hormone Health — 112

Bibliography — 117

Chapter 1
Does Your Metabolism Need a Reset?

Have you ever wondered why some women seem to eat whatever they want and stay effortlessly slim, while others can barely look at a piece of cake without gaining weight? It's easy to chalk it up to bad luck or genetics. The truth is more complicated—but far more empowering.

The secret lies in your metabolism, the engine that powers your body. While some people seem to have high-performance engines from birth, others might feel it's like driving a clunky old station wagon uphill. But here's the thing: you're not stuck with the engine you have. You can supercharge it, accelerate it, and get it humming like a dream.

This chapter is all about understanding your metabolism—how it works, why it might feel sluggish, and what you can do to turn it into a fat-burning machine. Once you understand the science, you'll see how small changes to what you eat and *when you eat* can make a world of difference.

What Is Metabolism, Really?

Metabolism is the process by which your body converts the food you eat into energy. Every time you eat a meal or take a breath, your body is working behind the scenes to extract energy from calories and keep your organs functioning. But here's the catch: not all metabolisms work at the same speed or efficiency.

Think of your metabolism as the engine of your body. Some engines burn through fuel (calories) with ease, while others are like outdated locomotives—slow, inefficient, and prone to storing excess fuel as fat.

The good news? You can rebuild and upgrade your engine, no matter where you're starting from.

Let's take a closer look at how this metabolic process works.

Metabolism covers all the chemical processes that turn the food you eat into energy, with various hormones at work—like insulin, which shuttles glucose into your cells, and ghrelin and leptin, which regulate hunger and fullness.

So imagine that inside your body there is a trendy nightclub called "Cells." This is where all the action happens that fuels your muscles, organs, and brain. Outside on the street—known as your bloodstream—glucose molecules (from the food you eat) are lining up, hoping to get in to Cells. Insulin stands at the door as the bouncer, holding the list and deciding who enters the club. When you eat a meal, more glucose (new partygoers) arrive on the street. If insulin is doing a good job, it waves in the right amount of glucose, so your cells get just the right amount of energy for a rocking dance floor. Any excess glucose gets sent to a "waiting room" — becoming glycogen in your liver and muscles— or, if that's full, to long-term storage — body fat.

For people with type 2 diabetes, their insulin isn't working properly —like a sleepy or overwhelmed bouncer—and it can't manage the crowd. The line (of blood sugar) grows as glucose lingers outside, and some partygoers get turned away or misdirected. Over time, this can lead to high blood sugar & "insulin resistance". By contrast, when insulin is alert and efficient, your cells maintain just the right balance—full of energy without creating a huge queue of sugar molecules desperately trying to get in.

After several hours without food—or during extended exercise—your body's readily available glucose and glycogen (short-term energy stored in muscles and liver) begin to deplete. Low blood sugar and reduced insulin levels send signals that you need more fuel. If no more food is consumed, the body turns to long-term storage and begins sourcing energy from fat.

This is when you have entered – **the fat burning zone**. (More on this in Chapters 3 & 4).

Muscle: The Metabolic MVP

If you've ever heard that muscle burns more calories than fat, it's not just fitness-industry hype—it's science. Muscle is metabolically active tissue, meaning it uses energy (calories) even when you're not moving. Fat, on the other hand, is like storage—it sits there, taking up space but not contributing much to the energy you burn.

A pound of muscle burns 6–10 calories a day, compared to just 2 calories for a pound of fat. That may not sound like much, but when you build even a few pounds of muscle, those extra calories burned can add up significantly over time.

Let's really take this in. **Muscle burns 3-5X more calories than fat** even while at rest.

Interestingly, this is one of the reasons it's recommended that men consume more calories per day than women. On average, men have more muscle mass and less body fat than women. So they can eat more calories per day without gaining fat.

It also explains why women can benefit tremendously from building muscle.

The Importance of Body Composition

Let's shift focus from the number on the scale to a more telling measurement: **body composition.**

Why Muscle Matters More Than Weight: Two women can weigh the same, but the one with more muscle will look leaner, feel stronger, and burn more calories at rest. This is why tracking your body fat percentage is far more valuable than obsessing over the scale.

The American Council on Exercise lists common body fat percentage ranges among women at different levels of fitness:

- Essential fat: 10–13%
- Athletes: 14–20%
- Fitness enthusiasts: 21–24%
- Healthy average: 25–31%
- Dangerously high (obese): 32% and over

A very rough and simple way to **estimate your body fat %** is to take your waist circumference in centimetres and divide by 2.7. For example, a 140lbs woman with a waist circumference of 80cm (about 32 inches) would have a body fat % of approximately 29-30%—in the healthy average range. However, a waist circumference of 87cm (or 34 inches) and over would result in a body fat % of 32% and be considered technically obese.

Many women fall into this category today. That's why it's so important to think about our body composition and take steps to keep it healthy.

Building muscle, therefore, isn't just about looking toned. It's about giving your body the tools it needs to burn calories more efficiently, stabilize blood sugar, and keep you fit and well. That's what metabolism is all about!

Your Metabolism as a Machine: What's Under the Hood?

Let's go back to the engine analogy. What are you carrying under your hood?

- **A High-Performance Engine:** This is someone with a balanced diet, a higher percentage of muscle mass, and an active lifestyle. Their body burns fuel efficiently, leaving little to store as fat.
- **An Overworked Locomotive:** This is someone whose metabolism is sluggish due to factors like low muscle mass, high body fat, irregular and unhealthy eating habits, or hormonal imbalances. Fuel that isn't burned off is stored for later use, often as fat.

What Happens As We Age

As we age, our metabolism naturally slows down—but that doesn't mean we're powerless.

Starting in your 30s, you lose about 3–8% of muscle mass per decade. By the 40s and 50s, this loss becomes more noticeable, reducing the body's overall calorie-burning capacity. Since muscle burns more calories than fat, losing it naturally leads to a slower metabolism and easier weight gain if diet and exercise habits remain unchanged.

In your 40s and 50s, a gradual drop in estrogen signals the transition from perimenopause into menopause. With less estrogen, the body begins storing more fat around the abdomen and less in the hips and thighs. Because estrogen also influences how our cells respond to insulin, lower levels can slow the metabolic rate and make fat burning more challenging. Progesterone levels also fall, disrupting the balance between estrogen and progesterone. This imbalance may lead to fluid retention, heightened appetite, and mood swings. At the same time, the thyroid, which helps regulate metabolism, can be thrown off by these hormonal changes, further complicating weight management.

Let's also be honest. Many of us don't hold ourselves to the same standards that we did when we were younger. We relax a little. We get comfortable. And so we should! Midlife often brings heavier demands—juggling career, family responsibilities, and personal goals. Chronic stress elevates cortisol levels, which in turn can trigger cravings for high-calorie "comfort foods" and prompt the body to store more fat, especially around the waistline. Hormonal fluctuations during this stage may also disturb sleep, creating a loop of poor rest, further stress, and an even slower metabolism. Long hours at a desk, poor sleep, and inconsistent eating habits can all drag your metabolism down.

The solution? Don't beat yourself up, nor throw in the towel. Create new habits and a life-long routine that you can stick with. One that will get your metabolism working for you, not against you.

What You'll Learn in This Book

Now that you have a clearer picture of how your metabolism works, you're ready to take control of it. This book will share:

1. How intermittent fasting can maximize your fat burning window and turn your metabolism into a high performance machine.
2. Which foods can provide the best fuel for your muscles and speed up your metabolic engine.
3. How timing meals with the right kind of exercise can super-charge fat burning and weight loss results.

You're Not Stuck With Your Metabolism

While some women seem gifted with an efficient metabolic engine from day one, no one is stuck with the metabolism they have. Your metabolism isn't static—it's a dynamic system that you can influence with the right habits and knowledge.

In the next chapter, we'll explore why traditional diet advice often falls short for modern women and how life's demands can sabotage even the best intentions. But don't worry—I'll also show you how to work around those challenges and reclaim control of your figure.

Chapter 2
How Life Sabotages Diet

For decades, our eating habits have been built around traditional work schedules— for example, eat breakfast at 7:00 a.m., lunch at noon, and dinner when we get home at night.

And by now, most people know the typical advice for a "healthy" diet: stick to whole, unprocessed foods, eat a high-protein breakfast and avoid big carb-heavy meals in the evening. You may also have heard this idea pulled together in the soundbite: "Eat like a king in the morning, a prince at lunch, and a pauper in the evening." Sounds simple enough, right? But in reality, life often has other plans. Between getting everyone out the door, juggling work responsibilities, and trying to squeeze in quality time with the family, most of us don't have the luxury of preparing perfect wholesome meals all the time. And this is where the problem begins.

For many women, especially those managing a household and a career, traditional diet advice is frustratingly impractical. The idea of cooking a nutritious high-protein breakfast at 7:00 a.m. before rushing off to work or packing school lunches just doesn't fit into real-life schedules. And what about family dinners? Eating a small meal at night while your family enjoys a full, satisfying dinner can feel isolating and unsustainable. This is why so many well-intentioned diets fail—they don't account for real-world demands.

The Disconnect Between Diet Advice and Real Life

Most diet plans are designed around an ideal schedule—one that assumes you have unlimited time, resources, and willpower to prepare and eat perfect meals. The reality, however, is much different. Here are some of the most common ways life gets in the way of even the best diet intentions.

Firstly, mornings are chaos. If you're someone who manages to prepare a high-protein breakfast for the whole family before school — that's great! But if you're like me, mornings are a mad dash to get everyone out the door. Many of us barely have time to do our makeup, let alone prepare a home-made protein-packed breakfast. Grabbing a sugary granola bar or calorific coffee becomes the norm. If this sounds familiar, you're not alone. The traditional "eat like a king at breakfast" advice doesn't fit into the reality of many women's lives.

Work schedules can also dictate eating patterns. Whether you're in back-to-back meetings or managing a demanding workload, we tend to eat whatever is convenient (often not the healthiest choice) or go too long without food, leading to intense hunger and overeating later.

Then there's the family to consider. The idea of eating "like a pauper" at dinner sounds good in theory, but in reality, sitting down for a hearty meal with loved ones is a treasured and meaningful part of the day. Restricting yourself while your family enjoys a balanced meal can feel like punishment.

And what about the weekend? Monday through Friday might be structured, but weekends introduce social events, family gatherings, and meals out—all of which make strict dieting difficult to maintain.

Stress, exhaustion, and emotional highs and lows can also make junk food all the more tempting. When willpower is drained at the end of the day, reaching for comfort food becomes second nature.

While some men can follow structured diet plans with fewer challenges, women's bodies and lifestyles are different. Our metabolism is more sensitive to stress, our hormonal cycles influence hunger and cravings, and we're often the ones responsible for feeding others—not just ourselves. Diet plans that don't consider these realities set women up for frustration.

Instead of working against life's natural rhythms, we need a way of eating that works *with* them. This is where the Brunch Yourself Thin method comes in—because it acknowledges real-life schedules and responsibilities while still supporting metabolic health and weight loss.

The Key to Success: A Sustainable, Flexible Plan

Rather than following unrealistic diet rules, the key to long-term success is to create a sustainable routine that fits your actual lifestyle. The Brunch Yourself Thin method is built on the idea that you can achieve lasting weight loss without giving up family dinners, obsessing over calories or food choices, or trying to force a morning routine that doesn't work for you. By shifting your first meal to a later brunch, and aligning exercise with optimal metabolic timing

(Chapter 11), you can work *with* your body to achieve your weight loss goals.

A Weight Loss Routine Designed for Women Today

For years, we've been eating around our traditional work schedules, but today, our lives look much different. The rise of flexible working means that many of us are no longer confined to rigid office hours. This shift presents **a golden opportunity**: we can design a weight loss routine that works with *real* life, rather than forcing ourselves to follow outdated meal schedules.

Instead of trying to build the perfect breakfast when you're rushed and distracted, what if you simply waited? What if, instead of grabbing a quick sugary fix, you allowed your body to ease into the day and saved your first meal for when you could actually prepare something more nutritious?

The Core Principle of This Book: An 8-Hour Eating Window Starting With Brunch.

The **Brunch Yourself Thin method** organises your day into the following simple routine:

1. **A High-Protein Brunch** – Instead of eating as soon as you wake up, you delay your first calories until mid-morning (around 10:30a.m.), allowing your body to operate in fat-burning mode for a few hours before refuelling with a protein-packed meal.
2. **Muscle-Building Exercise** – Midday is an ideal time for exercise with a quick 30-minute workout. This aligns with your body's natural metabolic rhythm and helps maximize energy usage from your first meal.

3. **A Light Lunch** – A small, nutrient-rich lunch around 1:00 or 1:30 p.m. replaces snacking. This will give your body more of what it needs to repair itself after a workout and keep energy steady without overloading your digestion.
4. **A Balanced Dinner** – Enjoy a full meal with your family at 6:00 p.m. without guilt. You don't need to eat like a "pauper" at night (or even skip dessert) —just keep portions reasonable and focus on whole, nutritious foods when you can.
5. **An Overnight Fast** – When dinner is over, it's time to close the kitchen and give your digestion a rest. Within four to six hours of your last meal, your body will enter its fat burning mode. Here is where all the benefits of intermittent fasting start to kick in. (More on that in the next Chapter.)

A Plan That Works for *Real* Life

Rather than following unrealistic diet rules, the key to long-term success is to create a routine that fits your actual lifestyle. The Brunch Yourself Thin method allows you to prioritize family meals without sacrificing weight loss goals and works whether you're a busy mom, a professional, or navigating midlife changes.

Now that we've laid out the foundation of this weight loss routine, the next chapters will dive deeper into meal timing, metabolic benefits, and how to customize this approach to suit your own lifestyle.

Chapter 3
Timing - The Secret Ingredient for a Faster Metabolism

Your metabolism doesn't just care about what you eat—it cares *when* you eat.

Your body has natural rhythms, and working with them instead of against them can dramatically improve how efficiently you burn calories. Here's two examples.

Insulin Sensitivity Peaks in the Morning: Your body is better at processing and storing nutrients earlier in the day. Eating nutritious meals in the morning helps prevent fat storage and stabilizes blood sugar levels.

The Body Turns to Fat for Energy When We Fast: As we saw in Chapter 1, the body runs on two types of fuel: carbohydrates (which are stored in your body as glycogen) and fat. When you eat throughout the day—especially meals loaded with carbs—your body primarily burns glycogen for energy. But when you take a break from eating, like during a fast, your glycogen stores begin to run low, and your body switches gears to burn fat instead.

Here's a detailed **timeline of what happens in your body after you consume a meal**, including digestion, blood sugar changes, energy storage, and fat metabolism:

0–30 Minutes: Digestion Begins

- As soon as food enters your mouth, enzymes in your saliva start breaking down carbohydrates.
- In the stomach, gastric acids begin digesting proteins and fats.
- Blood sugar starts to rise if the meal contains carbohydrates.

30 Minutes – 1 Hour: Peak Blood Sugar & Insulin Response

- Glucose from carbs enters the bloodstream, leading to an increase in blood sugar.
- The pancreas releases insulin to help shuttle glucose into your cells for energy or storage.
- If the meal was high in simple sugars, blood sugar spikes quickly. If it contained fiber, protein, or healthy fats, the rise is more gradual.

1 – 2 Hours: Energy Use & Nutrient Absorption

- Glucose is actively being used for energy or stored as glycogen in the liver and muscles.
- Amino acids from proteins are absorbed and used for muscle repair, enzyme production, and other bodily functions.
- Fat digestion and absorption continue at a slower pace, with fatty acids entering the bloodstream.

- If insulin levels were high, excess glucose starts getting stored in fat cells if energy demand is low.

3 – 4 Hours: Blood Sugar Returns to Normal

- Blood sugar and insulin levels start to decline as nutrients are distributed and used.
- If insulin was high (from a high-carb meal), this drop can sometimes lead to hunger and cravings.
- Fat burning is minimal, as the body is still using readily available glucose and glycogen.

4 – 6 Hours: Transition from Fed State to Fasted State

- Glycogen from the liver begins breaking down to maintain blood sugar levels.
- If insulin levels have dropped sufficiently, the body may start burning fat for energy.
- Hunger hormones (ghrelin) may begin rising, signalling the body to eat again.

6 – 12 Hours: Fat Burning Increases

- The body shifts more towards fat metabolism as glycogen stores become depleted.
- If no additional food is consumed, insulin remains low, and stored fat is broken down for energy.
- Ketone production may begin, depending on how long you've gone without eating and how much glycogen was stored initially.

12 – 16 Hours: Deep Fat Burning & Metabolic Shift

- Fat stores become the primary energy source as glycogen reserves are further depleted.
- Autophagy (cellular repair and regeneration) kicks in, where the body starts breaking down old, damaged cells.
- Insulin remains low, maximizing fat oxidation.
- Growth hormone levels increase, supporting muscle preservation and fat metabolism.

Beyond 16+ Hours: Extended Fasting Benefits

- If fasting continues, the body further enhances fat burning and ketone production.
- Autophagy intensifies, helping with anti-aging and cellular repair.
- Metabolic efficiency improves, making the body more adapted to burning fat as fuel.

This is where **Intermittent Fasting** comes into play—a simple yet powerful approach that allows your body to optimize energy use, burn fat more efficiently, and improve overall health.

Chapter 4
Making Intermittent Fasting Work for You

Fasting has been practiced for centuries, primarily for religious, cultural, and medical reasons. Many ancient civilizations, including those following Hinduism, Christianity, Islam, and Judaism, incorporated fasting into their spiritual traditions. In the early 20th century, medical researchers began exploring fasting as a therapeutic tool for obesity and metabolic health. By the 1960s, scientific interest grew, with studies investigating the effects of extended fasting periods ranging from one to fourteen days.

More recently, intermittent fasting has gained popularity as a modern health strategy, with various approaches such as alternate-day fasting, time-restricted eating, and the 5:2 diet emerging.

Intermittent fasting isn't about starving yourself; it's about structuring your eating window in a way that supports your metabolism and energy levels. Those who follow the strictest daily intermittent fasting schedule might fast for 18 or even 20 consecutive hours. However, a 16-hour fasting window is more than sufficient for your body to enter its fat-burning mode and deliver rapid and/or sustained weight loss.

In this plan, you'll follow a **16:8 fasting schedule**, meaning you fast for 16 hours and eat within an 8-hour window. The Brunch Yourself Thin method follows this structure:

- **10:30 AM – Brunch**
- **1:30 PM – Light Lunch**
- **6:00 PM – Dinner**

It's a simple concept: instead of eating from the moment you wake up until the moment you go to bed, you limit your eating window to a specific number of hours. Outside of this window, you're in a fasting state—allowing your body time to rest, repair, and shift into fat-burning mode.

If you're constantly snacking or eating late into the night, you may never give your body the chance to reach this fat-burning mode. By keeping your eating within a shorter time frame, you allow your body to fully shift into fat-burning mode during your fasting hours.

Why a 16-Hour Fast Maximizes Fat Burning

During fasting, your body goes through several metabolic changes that encourage fat loss:

1. Lower Insulin Levels – When you eat, insulin levels rise to help process glucose. When you fast, insulin levels drop, signalling the body to burn stored fat for energy.
2. Increased Human Growth Hormone (HGH) – Fasting

boosts HGH levels, which aid in muscle maintenance, fat burning, and overall metabolic function.
3. Fat Adaptation – Without a constant supply of food, your body shifts from burning sugar for energy to burning stored fat, making weight loss more efficient.

During the fasting period, your body doesn't have a steady stream of incoming calories, so it relies on stored energy—fat!

Other Benefits of Fasting for 16 Hours

Beyond fat loss, fasting offers a range of powerful health benefits:

Anti-Aging & Cellular Repair: During fasting, your body undergoes autophagy, a process where old and damaged cells are broken down and replaced with new, healthier cells. This has been linked to increased longevity and anti-aging effects.

Anti-Inflammatory Effects: Fasting reduces inflammation, which is a major contributor to chronic illnesses such as heart disease, diabetes, and autoimmune disorders.

Improved Brain Function: Studies suggest that fasting increases brain-derived neurotrophic factor (BDNF), a protein that supports brain health, memory, and cognitive function.

Better Digestion: Giving your digestive system a break for 16 hours helps improve gut health and can reduce bloating, sluggishness, and digestive discomfort.

Does Fasting Mean "No Coffee or Tea"?

Fasting means avoiding anything that triggers an insulin response or disrupts the metabolic benefits of fasting—but black coffee and unsweetened tea are completely fine. In fact, they can actually enhance fasting benefits by supporting fat metabolism, boosting mental clarity, and helping to curb appetite.

Black coffee contains zero calories and may increase fat oxidation, making it a great companion to intermittent fasting. However, adding milk, cream, sugar, or syrups will break your fast by introducing calories and triggering an insulin response. If you prefer something in your coffee, a tiny splash of unsweetened almond milk or MCT oil is less likely to disrupt fasting.

Most teas are also fasting-friendly, especially black & green Tea which contains caffeine and antioxidants that may enhance metabolism and fat burning. Oolong Tea may support fat oxidation and digestion. White Tea is a mild, antioxidant-rich option that can gently boost metabolism.

Herbal teas, like peppermint, chamomile, ginger, and rooibos, are naturally caffeine-free and offer additional digestive, anti-inflammatory, and relaxation benefits. They can help with hydration, gut health, and stress reduction—all of which support a successful fasting routine.

So the bottom line is: yes, you can drink coffee and tea while fasting—just avoid cream, sugar, and flavored syrups to maximize benefits. Herbal teas are an especially great option for hydration and digestive support during fasting hours.

Retraining Your Body

By adopting an 8 hour eating schedule, you're not just timing your meals—you're giving your body the opportunity to operate more efficiently and burn more fat. You're essentially **teaching your body to prioritize fat as a fuel source** rather than constantly using glucose or glycogen from recent meals. This is what will take your metabolic engine from an overworked locomotive to a high performance machine, and this reset is when serious weight loss begins.

In the next section, we'll break down how to build the perfect brunch to fuel your metabolism and set you up for success throughout the day.

Chapter 5
Building The Perfect Brunch

What Happens When We Eat an Ultra-Processed, High-Carb, or High-Sugar Meal?

Picture this: you wake up and reach for a sugary cereal or a processed breakfast bar. Within minutes, your body rapidly absorbs the simple carbohydrates, spiking your blood sugar. Your pancreas responds by releasing a surge of insulin, which helps shuttle glucose into your cells. But here's the problem—this quick spike is often followed by a rapid crash, leaving you feeling sluggish, hungry, and craving more sugar just an hour or two later.

Understanding the Glycemic Index and How It Affects Your Metabolism

Let's talk about something that's often misunderstood when it comes to food and metabolism: how different carbohydrates affect your blood sugar. You might have heard people talk about the glycemic index or glycemic load, but what do they really mean, and why should you care?

The **glycemic index is a ranking system for foods that contain carbohydrates**, but that doesn't mean it's only about things we traditionally call "carbs" like bread and pasta. It applies to any food that has digestible carbohydrates, including fruits, vegetables, legumes, and even dairy.

When we think of "carbs," we often picture things like rice, potatoes, and pasta. But carbohydrates are found in many whole foods, too—like bananas, apples, sweet potatoes, and milk. That's why these foods also have a glycemic index score. The glycemic index does not apply to foods that contain little to no carbohydrates, like meat, fish, eggs, or oils. That's why you won't see a GI score for a steak or an avocado.

Not all carbs behave the same way, however. Imagine your body is like a fireplace. When you add fuel to a fire, some things burn quickly, like paper, while others burn more slowly, like a thick log. In this analogy, different types of carbohydrates act like different fuels. Some cause a big burst of flames, while others keep a slow, steady burn going for hours. That's exactly what happens in your body when you eat different kinds of carbs.

The glycemic index (GI) is a way of measuring how fast a particular food raises your blood sugar. Foods that break down quickly and cause a rapid rise in blood sugar, like white bread or sugary cereal, have a high glycemic index. These are like throwing dry twigs into a fire—quick to burn, but they don't last long. On the other hand, foods that break down more slowly, like rolled oats, lentils, or sweet potatoes, have a lower glycemic index, meaning they provide a steady, sustained source of energy.

At first glance, it might seem like the glycemic index is all you need to know. But there's a catch. The glycemic index only tells you how quickly a food raises blood sugar, not how much of that food you're likely to eat in one sitting. That's where the glycemic load (GL) comes in.

Food	Glycemic Index (GI)	Glycemic Load (GL)
Sugary Cereal	75	42
White Pasta	64	25
White Rice	73	22
White Bread	75	20
Wholewheat Pasta	48	18
Brown Rice	55	16
Instant Oats	83	12
Steel-Cut Oats	53	7
Sweet Potato	63	14
Banana	51	13
Lentils	32	5
Strawberries	40	5
Blueberries	40	4
Watermelon	72	4
Greek Yogurt	11	3

Think of glycemic load as the real-world impact of a food on your blood sugar. A food might have a high glycemic index but a low glycemic load because you wouldn't normally eat enough of it to cause a big problem. For example, watermelon has a high glycemic index, but since it's mostly water and you'd have to eat a huge portion to cause a spike, its glycemic load is actually quite low. On the flip side, a big bowl of white rice has both a high glycemic index and a high glycemic load, meaning it will spike your blood sugar and keep it elevated for longer.

Why does this matter for metabolism? Your body is always trying to maintain balance. When you eat high-GI foods, your blood sugar spikes quickly, which prompts your pancreas to release a surge of insulin. Remember, insulin is the hormone that helps move sugar from your bloodstream into your cells, where it can be used for energy. But if this process happens too often—like when you eat a diet filled with high-GI, high-GL foods—your body can start to become resistant to insulin, making it harder to regulate blood sugar and increasing your risk of weight gain, energy crashes, and even metabolic disorders like type 2 diabetes.

On the other hand, when you eat lower-GI, lower-GL foods, you get a much more stable release of energy. Your blood sugar stays steady, your body doesn't have to pump out excessive insulin, and your metabolism hums along efficiently. This is why balancing your meals with fiber, protein, and healthy fats is so important—it slows down digestion and helps keep blood sugar levels in check.

A good way to think about this is to picture two people at a theme park. One person rushes to the biggest rollercoaster and experiences a thrilling, heart-pounding ride followed by an immediate drop and exhaustion. The other person takes a steady-paced stroll around the park, enjoying the attractions without the energy crashes. High-GI foods are like that rollercoaster—quick spikes and dramatic crashes—while low-GI foods provide a smooth and consistent source of energy, keeping you feeling good for longer.

So, does this mean you should never eat high-GI (carb heavy) foods?

I firmly believe that a life without these so-called "comfort foods" would be pretty miserable—and ultimately unsustainable for most of us. Also, it's completely unnecessary to give them up forever.

What really matters is:

a. How you balance high-GI, carb-heavy foods with lower-GI complements.
b. How often you eat them—moderation is key.
c. **When** you eat them—timing them within your 8 hour window can make all the difference.

When it comes to the Brunch Yourself Thin method, choosing lower-GI, protein and fiber-rich foods for your brunch—like eggs with avocado, steel-cut oats with nuts, or Greek yogurt with berries—will keep your metabolism running smoothly, i.e. you'll avoid the energy rollercoaster and keep cravings in check. (More on that in the next section.)

But if you're someone who thinks life isn't worth living without a bagel and cream cheese in the morning, I say go for it—just do it the smart way. Save it for brunch, balance it out by adding a side of protein—like smoked salmon or eggs—and pair it with an effective calorie-burning, muscle-building workout afterward. (In fact, if you've just finished an intense workout, a higher-GI food might actually be beneficial, as your muscles are primed to absorb that sugar for recovery.)

This way, you still get to enjoy the foods you love, but in a way that works with your metabolism, not against it. Overall, it's balancing your meals that matters more than just the glycemic index alone. If you've ever had a big bowl of pasta and felt hungry again an hour later, it's because a high-carb meal without protein or fat burns fast and leaves you craving more. But when you mix your carbs with protein—like eggs with toast, or chicken with brown rice—you get a steady, longer-lasting energy release instead of a sugar crash.

Fats also play a role, though in a different way. They don't spike blood sugar, but they affect insulin sensitivity over time. The right kinds of fats—like the ones in avocados, nuts, and olive oil—actually help improve metabolism and hormone balance. On the flip side, unhealthy fats—like trans fats found in processed foods—can do the opposite, making it harder for your body to regulate blood sugar properly.

Understanding the glycemic index and glycemic load doesn't mean you have to obsess over every bite of food. But being aware of how different foods affect your body helps you make smarter choices that support your metabolism and energy levels. And in the long run, that's what really makes a difference.

The 3Ps: Protein, Produce, and Portion Control

A well-balanced brunch follows the 3Ps:

1. **Protein**: The foundation of your meal, keeping you full and fuelling muscle maintenance.
2. **Produce**: Fiber-rich veggies or fruits add antioxidants, vitamins, and digestive benefits.
3. **Portion Control**: Eating enough to feel satisfied but not overstuffed, helping regulate energy intake throughout the day.

Why Do Experts Now Recommend a High-Protein Diet?

In contrast to a carb-heavy breakfast, a high-protein meal sets your metabolism up for success. Protein provides a steady source of energy, keeps you full longer, and helps preserve lean muscle mass, which is key for an efficient metabolism.

Modern research supports protein-rich meals for weight loss and metabolic health because protein has a high thermic effect: Your body burns more calories digesting protein than carbs or fat.

It is also the building block of muscle growth, and more muscle mass = a higher resting metabolic rate. (Remember this from Chapter 1 – muscle burns 3-5x more calories at rest than fat!)

Protein also helps keeps blood sugar stable. Unlike refined carbs, protein slows glucose absorption, preventing spikes and crashes. And it naturally curbs cravings. A protein-rich meal reduces ghrelin (the hunger hormone), keeping you satisfied for hours.

That's why building the perfect brunch around protein is the key to sustainable weight management.

How Much Protein Do We Need? (Men vs. Women)

The ideal protein intake depends on factors like age, activity level, and muscle mass goals. Here's a general guideline:

- Women: Aim for 0.8 to 1.2 grams of protein per kilogram of body weight (higher if strength training regularly).
- Men: Aim for 1.0 to 1.6 grams per kilogram of body weight (due to typically higher muscle mass).

For example, a 140-pound (63 kg) woman should aim for at least **50–90g of protein daily** depending on her activity level. For brunch, this translates to at least **20–30g of protein**—which can easily be achieved with eggs, natural Greek yogurt, cottage cheese, or lean meats.

There is also growing evidence that protein needs actually increase with age, especially for women over 50. Here's why:

1. Muscle Loss with Age (Sarcopenia). Starting around age 30, women naturally lose 3-8% of muscle mass per decade if they don't actively maintain it. By age 50-60, this

process accelerates, making protein intake even more critical.
2. Lower Efficiency in Protein Utilization. As we age, the body processes protein less efficiently, meaning older adults need slightly more protein per meal to trigger muscle protein synthesis. This means that a 60-year-old woman might need more protein than a 30-year-old woman to maintain the same muscle mass.
3. Higher Risk of Bone Loss. Protein supports bone health along with calcium and vitamin D. Older women (especially post-menopause) are at higher risk of osteoporosis, so keeping protein intake high helps maintain bone density and prevent fractures.

Here's a more detailed snapshot of the ideal amount of protein in grams an average sized (140lbs) woman should consume based on her age and activity level.

Age Group	Sedentary	Active and/or Strength Training
20-34	50g	75-90g
35-45	50g	75-90g
46-55	55g	80-95g
56-65	65g	80-95g
65+	65g	80-95g

The Best Sources of Protein to Fuel Your Metabolic Engine

Lean Protein: Helps sustain energy and keeps you full longer. The best options include:

- Grilled chicken, turkey, or fish
- Eggs or egg-based dishes
- Tofu or tempeh for plant-based eaters

- Greek yogurt or cottage cheese

	Protein (g)	Carbohydrates (g)	Fiber (g)	Saturated Fat (g)
Eggs (2)	13g	1g	0g	3.3g
Grilled Chicken	31g	0g	0g	1.0g
Turkey Breast	29g	0g	0g	0.7g
Fish (Salmon)	25g	0g	0g	3.2g
Tofu	8g	2g	1.9g	0.7g
Tempeh	19g	9g	1.5g	2.5g
Greek Yogurt (Plain, 2%)	10g	4g	0g	3.0g
Cottage Cheese (Low-fat)	12g	3g	0g	2.6g
Parma Ham (Prosciutto)	26g	0g	0g	6.3g
Bacon (Crispy)	37g	1g	0g	14g
Pork Sausage (Grilled)	18g	2g	0g	7.5g
Chorizo	24g	2g	0g	9g

Pork-based breakfast items like bacon, sausage, chorizo, and Parma ham are undeniably high in protein, making them an appealing choice for a protein-focused diet. However, they also come with significant amounts of saturated fat and sodium, which can be counterproductive if consumed frequently.

Many processed pork products contain 6-14g of saturated fat per 100g, which can contribute to increased LDL ("bad") cholesterol levels and a higher risk of heart disease when consumed in excess. Cured meats like bacon and Parma ham also contain large amounts of added salt, which can lead to water retention, bloating, and elevated blood pressure over time.

Instead, choose leaner pork cuts (like pork loin or tenderloin) over heavily processed versions. Limit bacon, sausages, and cured meats to occasional indulgences rather than daily staples. Pair pork products with fiber-rich vegetables to help counteract their effects on digestion and cholesterol.

While pork can be a protein-rich addition to meals, prioritizing leaner protein sources like chicken, fish, eggs, and plant-based proteins will offer better long-term benefits for metabolism and overall health.

Legumes: are also a great source of protein especially for vegans or vegetarians, though they are relatively high in carbohydrates compared to animal-based protein sources.

	Protein (g)	Carbohydrates (g)	Fiber (g)
Lentils	9g	20g	8g
Chickpeas	8.9g	27g	7.4g
Black Beans	8.9g	22g	7.5g
Kidney Beans	7.0g	21g	8.0g
Pinto Beans	7.0g	22g	7.0g
Green Peas	5g	15g	5.5g
Edamame (Soybeans)	11g	9g	5g

Non-Starchy Vegetables: These provide fiber, vitamins, and minerals without excess carbs.

- Leafy greens (spinach, kale, arugula, romaine)
- Cruciferous veggies (broccoli, cauliflower, Brussels sprouts)
- Cucumbers, bell peppers, or zucchini

Healthy Fats: Keeps you satiated and helps with hormone regulation.

- Avocado slices or guacamole

- Olive oil dressing on a salad
- Nuts and seeds (almonds, walnuts, chia, flaxseed)
- Cheese (in moderation)

Other Smart Carbs (Optional, Based on Your Activity Level):

If you plan to have an active day or a tough workout, adding a small serving of whole grains can provide extra energy without causing sugar spikes. Examples:

- Quinoa, brown rice or sweet potatoes.
- A typical bowl of porridge oats (40g dry, cooked with water) provides approximately 5 grams of protein and 24 grams of carbohydrates.

Home Made Protein Smoothies are another easy and convenient way to get in an early dose of protein for brunch. Be sure to choose a protein powder without any artificial sweeteners. A good choice will include a natural sweetener like Stevia as well as other beneficial ingredients like Vitamin B, Magnesium, and Omega 3.

Stevia is natural – It's derived from the Stevia plant, making it a better alternative to artificial sweeteners like aspartame or sucralose. Unlike sugar, Stevia has zero calories and zero GI, so it doesn't spike blood sugar or insulin, making it fasting-friendly and good for weight loss. Some protein powders use sugar alcohols (like maltitol or sorbitol), which can cause bloating or digestive discomfort. Stevia is usually easier on the stomach. And there's no strong evidence that Stevia negatively affects metabolism or gut health when consumed in moderation.

The appendix of this book features delicious smoothie recipes and a sample 7 day meal plan for more inspiration. But I want to emphasis again, this very important point:

You do not need to follow an ideal, optimally balanced, whole food diet every single day for the Brunch Yourself Thin method to work.

If you want to have left-overs from last night's dinner—that's okay!

Or if you want to keep things simple and just have the same scrambled eggs for brunch every morning, I won't hold it against you! Particularly if you're at low risk for high cholesterol. In fact, recent research suggests the cholesterol in food has far less impact on blood cholesterol than previously thought. The Mayo Clinic notes that while eggs do contain cholesterol, their consumption doesn't necessarily raise cholesterol levels in the blood for most people. However, for those with genetic predispositions to high cholesterol, excessive egg consumption may slightly increase LDL (the "bad" cholesterol).

The real culprit behind heart disease isn't necessarily dietary cholesterol—it's ultra-processed foods, excessive sugar, and trans fats.

At the end of the day, **consistency beats perfection**. It's better to have the same simple, high-protein meal every morning than to stress about (and ultimately fail,) making the perfect, varied, whole foods diet.

Why Fruit is Contentious: The Pros & Cons

Some people avoid fruit, particularly strict followers of low-carb or keto diets, due to its natural sugar content. The concern is that fructose—a sugar found in fruit—may be directly converted to fat as well as spiking blood sugar (and contribute to insulin resistance if consumed in excess.)

Fructose and glucose are both simple sugars (monosaccharides), but they are processed differently in the body. Let's break it down step by step.

When you consume table sugar (sucrose)—found in fruit, processed foods, and sugary drinks—your body splits it into two simpler sugars:

- **Glucose** (50%)
- **Fructose** (50%)

Your body treats these two sugars very differently, which is why excessive fructose intake can have different metabolic effects than glucose.

How Glucose is Processed

Glucose is the body's primary energy source. When you eat glucose-containing foods (like bread, rice, potatoes, or fruit), glucose enters the bloodstream and raises blood sugar levels.

Insulin is released by the pancreas to help move glucose into cells, where it's used for energy or stored as glycogen in the liver and muscles. (Chapter 1).

Every cell in your body can directly use glucose for energy.

How Fructose is Processed

Fructose is metabolized differently than glucose because it is handled exclusively by the liver (unlike glucose, which is used by all cells).

When fructose enters the liver:

1. It doesn't immediately raise blood sugar the way glucose does because insulin does not regulate it directly.
2. The liver converts some fructose into glucose, which can then enter the bloodstream.
3. Any **excess fructose is converted directly into fat** if not needed for immediate energy. This process can contribute to fat accumulation in the liver and, in extreme cases, non-alcoholic fatty liver disease (NAFLD).
4. Fructose metabolism also produces uric acid, which has been linked to inflammation, high blood pressure, and gout.

Key Differences Between Fructose and Glucose

Feature	Glucose	Fructose
How it enters the bloodstream	Directly absorbed, raises blood sugar	Must be processed by the liver first
Insulin response	Triggers insulin release	Does not trigger insulin directly
Primary use	Immediate energy for cells	Mostly converted to fat or glucose in the liver
Fat storage potential	Lower (if burned for energy or stored as glycogen)	Higher (if consumed in excess, contributes to liver fat)
Health impact (excess consumption)	Can cause insulin resistance over time	Linked to fatty liver, high triglycerides, and metabolic issues

Does This Mean Fruit is Bad?

Not at all! Whole fruit is very different from added sugars.

Natural fruit contains fiber, water, and essential vitamins that slow down the absorption of fructose, preventing spikes in blood sugar. The problem arises with high-fructose corn syrup (HFCS) and excessive added sugars found in processed foods and sugary drinks.

These deliver large amounts of fructose quickly, overloading the liver and increasing fat production.

But there's more to the case for fruit. Fruit is a key source of antioxidants, which fight inflammation and promote healthy skin. It also provides essential vitamins and minerals that processed low-carb alternatives lack.

So should you eat fruit? The answer depends on your goals and how your body responds to it. For most people, whole fruits (not fruit juices) are a beneficial addition—especially when eaten alongside protein to prevent blood sugar spikes.

The Best Way to Eat ANY Sugar: With a Meal

If you enjoy sweet foods, timing matters. Eating fruit or sugary foods with a balanced meal—rather than on an empty stomach—helps prevent sharp blood sugar spikes and insulin swings. Here's why:

1. Protein and fiber slow digestion, reducing how quickly sugar enters the bloodstream.
2. Fat helps stabilize glucose levels, keeping energy steady.
3. A steady blood sugar response minimizes the likelihood of energy crashes and sugar cravings.

So in practice, having a piece of chocolate after a meal is far better than eating it alone as a snack, which could spike blood sugar and lead to hunger soon after.

Summing Up:

Here is a useful table summarising which foods provide the best fuel to speed up our metabolism:

Food	Metabolic Benefit
Protein-Rich Foods (Eggs, Fish, Lean Meat, Greek Yogurt)	High thermic effect, supports muscle growth, increases calorie burn
Green Tea & Coffee	Boosts fat oxidation, increases calorie burning, mild appetite suppressant
Chili Peppers & Spicy Foods	Capsaicin boosts thermogenesis, reduces appetite, increases fat oxidation
Whole Grains & Fiber-Rich Foods (Oats, Quinoa, Brown Rice, Legumes)	Requires more energy to digest, stabilizes blood sugar, keeps you full longer
Healthy Fats (Avocados, Nuts, Olive Oil, Fatty Fish)	Supports hormone balance, provides long-lasting energy, reduces inflammation
Apple Cider Vinegar	Improves insulin sensitivity, enhances fat burning, reduces appetite
Dark Chocolate (85%+ Cocoa)	Contains caffeine & polyphenols, improves insulin sensitivity, boosts energy
Water	Cold water increases calorie burn, supports digestion, prevents overeating

And by structuring your brunch around high-quality protein, fiber-rich produce, and mindful portions, you'll stabilize your metabolism and fuel your body properly. By combining any sweet foods, ideally whole fruits (but even chocolate ;) with a balanced meal, you'll maintain a stable blood sugar for your optimal metabolic engine.

Chapter 6
A Light & Later Lunch... Replaces Snacking

After your protein-packed brunch and mid-day workout (which we'll cover in Chapters 10 & 11), lunch plays a crucial role in keeping your metabolism steady and preventing the energy dips that lead to snacking. The goal isn't to have a huge, heavy meal but rather a light, nutrient-dense feed that sustains you until dinner without triggering cravings or afternoon sluggishness.

A well-balanced lunch should provide steady energy without causing a crash, be satisfying but not overly filling, keeping you alert and productive. And include protein, fiber, and healthy fats to prevent hunger before dinner.

What to Eat for Lunch

Your lunch should focus on quality over quantity. Instead of grabbing a processed sandwich, a sugary yogurt, or a quick snack bar, aim for whole, minimally processed foods.

Example Lunch Ideas:

1. Hearty lentil soup with wholegrain bread.
2. Egg Omelette with cherry tomatoes, feta and a raw green juice.
3. Mixed greens and a sprinkle of feta cheese.
4. Salmon with roasted veggies and a drizzle of tahini dressing.
5. Grilled chicken salad with olive oil dressing and avocado.
6. Greek yogurt & nuts with a side of cucumber slices and hummus.

AGAIN... Timing is Key.

By lunching slightly later than usual, we close the gap with dinner and make it less likely that we'll cave to mid-afternoon snacking.

The Problem with Snacking

Many diets fail because of mindless snacking. **The more often you eat, the more frequently your body releases insulin, making it harder to burn stored fat.**

The common snacking traps:

- Emotional eating: Reaching for food out of boredom, stress, or habit rather than true hunger.
- Sugary quick fixes: Processed snack bars, flavored yogurts, or crackers can create an energy spike, followed by a crash that leaves you craving more.
- Unconscious grazing: Grabbing handfuls of nuts, chips, or bites of leftovers throughout the afternoon adds up quickly.

Why Replacing Snacks with a Light Lunch Works

By eating a satisfying, balanced lunch, later in the day, you prevent the blood sugar crashes that lead to afternoon cravings. Instead of constantly spiking insulin with small snacks throughout the day, you give your body time to stabilize, making it easier to tap into stored fat for energy.

If you're used to snacking, this shift might take a few days to adjust. When 4:00p.m. rolls around – choose a black coffee or herbal tea instead. And once your body adapts, you'll feel more energized, focused, and in control of your appetite without the need for constant grazing.

If you must snack—you guessed it—snack on protein.

But, remember...

By making a light, late, protein-rich lunch your standard instead of relying on snacks, you'll naturally curb cravings and create a steady energy flow for the rest of the day. Next, we'll dive into how to enjoy a balanced, satisfying dinner without undoing your progress.

Chapter 7
The Golden Rules of Evening

While the right brunch sets us up for success, it's our evening habits that can make or break our metabolic efficiency. Evenings are often where we face the most temptation—and if we are too strict, we set ourselves up for failure.

Why the "Eat Like a Pauper" Advice Doesn't Work for Real Women

Many diet programs encourage people to "eat like a king at breakfast, a prince at lunch, and a pauper at dinner." The idea is that front-loading calories earlier in the day helps with energy levels and weight management. But while this advice may work in theory, it doesn't fit into real life for most women.

Here's why:

Family Dinner is a Non-Negotiable – For many women, dinner is the one meal where everyone gathers. Trying to eat a small, light meal while the rest of the family enjoys a satisfying, hearty dinner is miserable and unsustainable.

Evenings Are for Relaxing & Connecting – A shared evening meal with friends bolsters our spirits and supports our mental health. You don't want to be the person who orders a tiny salad while everyone else is tucking into something delicious.

Overly Restrictive – A restrictive meal at dinner can lead to frustration and later snacking, which defeats the purpose of the diet.

Instead of forcing a tiny, unsatisfying meal at night, it's far more effective in the long term to eat a well-balanced dinner that aligns with real-life routines.

Family Dinners Nourish More Than Just The Body

Sitting down for dinner together as a family isn't just about eating —it's a daily ritual that strengthens bonds, provides structure, and teaches children the importance of eating well-balanced, nutritious meals. Research shows that families who eat together tend to make healthier food choices, and children exposed to home-cooked meals are more likely to develop a positive relationship with food.

Dinner is also a time to enjoy real food without distractions, savoring meals rather than eating mindlessly in front of a screen. By making small but intentional choices, we can transform family favorites into nutrient-rich meals that support our health goals while still being delicious and satisfying.

How to Modify Family Favorites for Better Balance

You don't need to prepare separate meals to eat healthily. Instead, small tweaks can improve the nutritional balance of classic family dishes. Here are a few easy swaps:

1. Spaghetti Bolognese with a Side Salad
   - Swap white pasta for whole wheat or lentil pasta for extra fiber and protein.
   - Add grated zucchini or mushrooms to the Bolognese sauce for extra nutrients.
   - Serve with a side salad instead of garlic bread to balance the meal with greens.
2. Roast Chicken, Potatoes, and Colorful Veggies
   - Opt for roasting potatoes with the skin on to increase fiber.
   - Include a variety of colorful veggies to maximize vitamins and minerals.
   - Swap store-bought gravy for a homemade version to reduce unnecessary additives.
3. Cottage Pie with Sweet Potato Mash
   - Use lean ground beef or turkey to lower saturated fat.
   - Mash sweet potatoes with regular potatoes for added antioxidants.
   - Serve with a side of steamed carrots or peas for extra fiber and color.
4. Corn Tacos with Shredded Pork, Black Beans, Peppers & Onions
   - Use corn tortillas instead of flour for a more nutrient-dense base.
   - Add black beans for plant-based protein and fiber.
   - Load up on sautéed peppers and onions for extra vitamins and flavor.
5. 5-Bean Veggie Chili with Brown Rice
   - A great plant-based meal packed with protein and fiber.
   - Use brown rice or quinoa instead of white rice for better blood sugar control.

    - Top with Greek yogurt instead of sour cream for extra protein.
  6. Other Easy Balanced Dinner Ideas:
     - Salmon with Roasted Vegetables and Quinoa
     - Chicken Stir-Fry with Brown Rice & Broccoli
     - Homemade Burgers with a Lettuce Wrap Instead of a Bun
     - Grilled Steak with Asparagus & Baked Potato

Making swaps like these can accelerate your weight loss progress. However if you're dealing with picky eaters and just want to keep things simple–that's fine too. You will still lose weight on this program because you're establishing so many other metabolic-positive habits.

Yes, You Can Have Dessert!

Many people think they need to cut out sweets entirely to be healthy, but the key is eating them at the right time and in the right amounts. In Chapter 8, we already talked about how sweet foods, like dessert, when enjoyed as part of a meal, has a lesser impact on blood sugar because the protein, fiber, and healthy fats from dinner slow the absorption of sugar.

But let's also think about portion sizes. At the end of a meal, we're already feeling quite full and satisfied, so we're **more likely to opt for smaller portions** of our favourite treats.

Good dessert options include:

- Dark chocolate & nuts
- Homemade banana ice cream (frozen banana blended with almond milk)

- Baked apples with cinnamon

However, even if you want to really indulge, on a rich chocolate mousse for example (my favourite ;) the key is to enjoy treats like this in moderation—and to eat them as part of your meal, not as a separate snack later.

The No-Snacking Rule

Your body's metabolism is naturally slower at night, so eating large amounts before bed can lead to more fat storage.

One of the most common pitfalls in weight management is **mindless snacking after dinner**. If you've had a well-balanced meal at 6:00pm, your body shouldn't need more food before bed. However, habits, boredom, or emotional eating often lead to unnecessary late-night snacking, which can disrupt digestion, blood sugar balance, and sleep quality.

What we want to avoid at all costs is the scenario where we start the evening full of good intentions, have a small dinner at 6:00p.m., and then raid the snack cupboard a few hours later, consuming an entire packet of cookies. As we saw in previous chapters, doing so would flood the body with glucose and fructose, and take you out of the fat-burning zone.

<u>**Nothing will sabotage your metabolism more than regular late night sugar binges.**</u>

To avoid snacking in the evenings:

- Eat a fulfilling, well-balanced dinner.
- Drink herbal tea to signal the end of eating for the day.

- Brush your teeth after dinner to mentally "close the kitchen."

Your 16-Hour Fast Begins

With dinner finished and the kitchen closed, your fasting period begins. Over the next few hours, your body will shift into digestive rest mode, allowing insulin levels to drop and fat-burning mechanisms to activate. By the time you wake up, your body will have entered a fasted state, where it begins to rely more on stored energy for fuel.

During this time:

- Insulin levels decrease, allowing the body to shift from storing energy to burning fat.
- Growth hormone increases, which helps with muscle preservation and fat metabolism.
- Cellular repair processes like autophagy (removal of damaged cells) begin.

This overnight fast helps reset metabolism, improve insulin sensitivity, and optimize fat burning, setting you up for success the next day. All you have to do is avoid late-night snacking and let your body do its work!

Recapping the Golden Rules

The golden rules of evening are: enjoy a balanced family dinner, and swap snacks for fasting to begin your metabolic reset. Dinner should be nutritious, satisfying, and family-friendly—not a battle between eating "clean" and enjoying food. By making simple adjustments to your favorite meals, you can create an evening routine that supports both your health goals and your family's well-being. And by following the no-snacking rule, you can reset your metabolism through the proven power of intermittent fasting.

Chapter 8
Cheat Days

Cheat days are a hot topic in the world of dieting. Some people swear by them as a mental reset, while others worry they'll undo their progress. In the context of intermittent fasting and metabolic health, cheat days aren't just about indulging—they can actually serve a biological purpose when used correctly.

At its core, intermittent fasting works by regulating insulin, increasing fat oxidation, and improving metabolic flexibility. But prolonged fasting—**especially when combined with calorie restriction**—can cause the body to adapt by lowering metabolism and slowing fat loss. That's the opposite of what we want! This is because if you stay in a caloric deficit for too long, your body may reduce energy expenditure to conserve resources. A well-planned cheat day **reminds your body that it's not starving**, keeping your metabolism active and responsive.

Prolonged fasting and calorie restriction can also lower leptin levels, increasing hunger and making fat loss harder. A higher-calorie day can boost leptin, helping you feel satisfied and supporting continued weight loss.

What's more, if you've been following low-carb meals, your glycogen (stored carbohydrates in muscles and liver) may be running low. A cheat day with some extra smart carbs can refuel your muscles, improving energy, recovery, and workout performance.

Ultimately, the biggest reason diets fail? They feel too restrictive. Knowing you can enjoy your favorite foods without guilt makes it easier to stick to your routine long-term.

How to Have a Smart Cheat Day Without Undoing Progress

Not all cheat days are created equal! The key is balance—you can indulge without going overboard and triggering negative metabolic effects.

- Stick to an 8-Hour Eating Window – Even on a cheat day, fasting before and after indulgence helps regulate insulin and control blood sugar spikes.
- Include Protein to Reduce Overeating – Protein slows digestion and prevents a cheat from turning into an all-day binge.
- Use It as a Mental Reset, Not an Excuse – A cheat day isn't about stuffing yourself sick—it's about enjoying food without guilt and moving forward the next day.

The 80/20 Rule

If what you're putting into your body is wholesome and nutritious 80% of the time, you can certainly achieve a healthy body and beautiful figure. Indulging on heavy carbs and sugary treats 20% of the time is a realistic balance given the modern world we live in.

The great thing about the habitual weight loss routine recommended in this book is that it allows you to still eat the foods you love and achieve your goals.

So, Let's Cheat!

A cheat day can be a helpful tool for both metabolic and psychological reasons. For those on restricted calories, it keeps metabolism humming. And for everyone else, it prevents diet burnout and makes weight loss sustainable rather than restrictive.

The best approach? Enjoy your indulgence, move on, and get back to your routine the next day—no guilt, no stress.

Chapter 9
Bonus Diet Hack

Stop Consuming Mindless Liquid Calories!

You might be carefully watching what you eat, making smart choices, and following the Brunch Yourself Thin method—but if you're drinking the wrong things, you could still be sabotaging your progress without even realizing it. Many people overlook liquid calories, but they can add up quickly and lead to unwanted weight gain, blood sugar spikes, and sluggish metabolism. The good news? This is one of the easiest diet fixes you can make!

Why Liquid Calories Are a Problem

Unlike solid foods, liquid calories don't provide the same feeling of fullness. Your body processes drinks differently than whole foods, meaning you could consume hundreds of extra calories without feeling satisfied. Sugary beverages also cause rapid blood sugar spikes, leading to insulin crashes, cravings, and energy dips later in the day.

Calorie Counting Example: How Beverages Can Add Up

Let's look at how much hidden sugar and calories can come from daily drinks:

Beverage	Calories (per serving)	Sugar Content
Regular Soda (12 oz)	150	39g
Flavored Latte (16 oz)	250-400	30-50g
Fruit Juice (12 oz)	180	42g
Sweetened Iced Tea (16 oz)	180	44g
Sports Drink (20 oz)	140	36g
Energy Drink (16 oz)	200	54g
Wine (5 oz)	120	1-2g
Beer (12 oz)	150	0g
Mixed Cocktail	200-400	Varies
Protein Shake (store-bought)	200-300	20-30g

Drinking just one of these per day can add 1,000+ extra calories in a week—without you even realizing it! That's an entire extra day's worth of food in calorie equivalents.

Better Choices: Low-Calorie & Metabolism-Friendly Drinks

Instead of sugary, high-calorie beverages, opt for drinks that hydrate and support fat loss:

- Water – The ultimate zero-calorie drink.
- Black Coffee or Espresso – Boosts metabolism without added sugar or cream.
- Herbal or Green Tea – Provides antioxidants and supports digestion.
- Sparkling Water with Lemon – A refreshing, flavored alternative to soda.
- Homemade Smoothies – Blend whole fruits, greens, and protein instead of store-bought versions.
- Electrolyte Water (Unsweetened) – Replenishes hydration without unnecessary sugars.

Cocktails vs. Chocolate: Which is the Bigger Sugar Bomb?

Many people associate sugar and extra calories with sweet treats and desserts, but they don't always consider how much sugar is lurking in their drinks—especially alcoholic ones. Take a standard milk chocolate bar, which has about 230 calories and 24 grams of sugar. Now compare that to a Piña Colada, which packs 400 calories and 60 grams of sugar—more than double the sugar in a chocolate bar! Margaritas, too, can have 36 grams of sugar, making it just as much of a dessert as a sweet treat.

Eye-opening isn't it? Next time you're thinking of ordering a third margarita, imagine you're ordering a third dessert instead!

Skinny Cocktails: Smarter Alcohol Choices

Alcohol itself isn't necessarily the enemy—it's what you mix it with that often causes the damage. Many traditional cocktails are loaded with sugary syrups, fruit juices, and sweet mixers, which spike insulin levels and add hundreds of unnecessary calories. The solution? Opt for "skinny" cocktail alternatives that cut out the excess sugar while still letting you enjoy a drink.

Instead of a Margarita with triple sec and sweet syrup, go for a Skinny Margarita with fresh lime juice, tequila, and a splash of soda water. Instead of a Gin & Tonic made with regular tonic (which contains as much sugar as a soda), switch to a Gin & Diet Tonic or a Vodka Soda with lime. Small swaps like these can make a major difference in your calorie and sugar intake without sacrificing your social life.

Small Change, Big Impact

Cutting back on liquid calories is one of the easiest, fastest ways to reduce calorie intake without feeling deprived. Simply swapping sugary drinks for water, black coffee, or herbal tea can make a huge difference in weight loss, blood sugar control, and energy levels. Try making this small shift, and watch how much better you feel—without even changing what's on your plate!

In the next chapter, we'll dive deeper into exercise and see how the right kind of exercise at the right time can rapidly accelerate weight loss and create the lean, toned figure you've always dreamed of.

Chapter 10
The Right Exercise Can Supercharge Your Results

Let's clear up a common misconception—that if you want to lose fat, you need to do to lots of cardio. Instead, a more efficient and effective strategy is to **focus on building muscle**. Why? Because muscle is metabolically active, meaning the more muscle you have, the more calories your body burns—even when you're just sitting around. That's right—building muscle means your body turns into a fat-burning machine, even when you're resting on the couch.

Why Building Muscle Helps Burn More Fat

Remember our metabolic engine from Chapter 1. A body with more muscle mass is like a high-performance sports car, burning fuel (calories) more efficiently. A body with less muscle is more like an old station wagon—slow to burn energy. If you want to rev up your metabolism, strength training is key.

Here's what happens when you build muscle:

- Muscle increases your resting metabolic rate (RMR) – This means your body naturally burns more calories throughout the day, even when you're not working out.
- Strength training prevents muscle loss while losing weight – If you're losing weight without lifting weights, you're likely losing muscle too, which can slow down your metabolism.
- More muscle = better fat oxidation – Muscle tissue improves the body's ability to process and burn fat for energy.

So if your goal is to lose fat and keep it off, strength training to build muscle should be a non-negotiable part of your routine.

Addressing the Fear of "Bulking Up"

One of the biggest concerns many women have about strength training is the fear of getting "bulky." So, let's set the record straight.

Building a bulky, muscular physique does not happen by accident. Women have far lower levels of testosterone than men, which makes it much harder to develop large, heavily muscled frames. The type of training recommended in this book—moderate strength training combined with smart nutrition and intermittent fasting—will not make you bulky. Instead, it will help you build a toned, sculpted, and leaner body.

To truly "bulk up," you would need to do the following:

- Eat in a calorie surplus, consuming significantly more calories than you burn.

- Lift extremely heavy weights with low reps, targeting hypertrophy.
- Follow a highly specialized training program designed for muscle mass gain.

Since this book recommends a combination of strength training, metabolic conditioning, and controlled nutrition, the result will be a lean, firm, and defined physique—not bulk.

If anything, strength training helps create that "toned" look most women desire. The reason? Tone comes from muscle definition, which becomes more visible as body fat decreases. By increasing muscle without increasing fat, your body will appear leaner, stronger, and more sculpted.

Rather than making you look bulky, strength training is your secret weapon for a fit, feminine, and empowered body.

How Do Muscles Grow

As we discussed in Chapter 5, Protein is the building block of muscle growth. Every time you engage in strength training or resistance exercise, your muscles experience tiny tears (microtears) at the cellular level. This is called muscle protein breakdown (MPB)—a natural process that occurs during exercise. It is completely normal and necessary for muscle growth—but they require repair and rebuilding. This is where protein plays a crucial role.

Protein is made up of amino acids, which act like building blocks for your muscles. Your body pulls amino acids from food (or muscle tissue if protein intake is low) to repair and rebuild these fibers.

After exercise, your body shifts into muscle protein synthesis (MPS)—a process where amino acids from protein are used to repair and rebuild muscle fibers stronger and thicker than before. To gain muscle, muscle protein synthesis must exceed muscle protein breakdown—which is why consuming enough protein is essential. Without adequate protein, your body can't fully repair the muscle damage from workouts, leading to slower progress, increased soreness, and even potential muscle loss.

If your protein intake is too low over an extended period, your body may struggle to access enough amino acids to repair damaged muscle fibers. In extreme cases, it may catabolize existing muscle tissue (break it down) to supply the necessary amino acids for recovery. However, this is more likely to happen if you're consistently undereating protein and calories or you're doing intense workouts with inadequate workout nutrition. In that case, your body is in a prolonged catabolic state (fasting too long after exercise without protein intake).

To prevent this, aim to consume protein throughout the day rather than relying solely on one large meal. A well-balanced diet will support muscle repair and growth without breaking down existing muscle tissue.

So REMEMBER: Muscle growth is a balance between exercise and proper nutrition. Protein provides the essential amino acids your body needs to repair, rebuild, and strengthen muscle tissue after workouts. **Without enough protein, your body struggles to recover, limiting muscle gains** and increasing the risk of muscle breakdown.

Strength Training Is the Key To Muscle Growth

Strength training, also called resistance training, involves exercises that challenge your muscles using resistance. This can come from your own body weight, free weights, resistance bands, or gym machines. The goal is to stimulate muscle growth, improve strength, and enhance overall metabolic efficiency.

Here are some of the best strength training exercises, categorized by muscle group:

Full-Body Strength Training Routine (Beginner-Friendly):

1. Squats – Works legs, glutes, and core. Start with bodyweight squats, then progress to dumbbells or a barbell.
2. Push-Ups – Strengthens chest, shoulders, and triceps. Modify by starting on knees or against a wall.
3. Deadlifts – Engages hamstrings, glutes, lower back, and core. Begin with light weights to master form.
4. Lunges – Targets legs and glutes while improving balance.
5. Planks – Strengthens the core, shoulders, and back. Try variations like side planks or plank-to-push-up.
6. Dumbbell Shoulder Press – Builds shoulder strength and stability.
7. Pull-Ups (or Assisted Pull-Ups) – Develops upper-body strength, focusing on back and arms.
8. Rows (Dumbbell or Barbell) – Strengthens back muscles and improves posture.

If you're new to strength training, start with 3-4 sessions per week, performing 8-12 repetitions per exercise for 2-3 sets. As you get stronger, gradually increase resistance by adding weights or resistance bands.

Access to a gym is ideal but certainly not necessary. Thousands of free strength training workout videos are available on Youtube and can be done in the comfort of your living room.

The "After Burn Effect"

The "after burn effect" is a popular term for the scientific phenomenon known as Excess Post-Exercise Oxygen Consumption (EPOC). After an intense workout, your body continues to consume more oxygen than normal in order to return itself to a resting state. Because oxygen consumption is tied to energy expenditure, this means you'll continue burning calories at an elevated rate even after your workout ends.

EPOC refers to the extra calories you burn after exercise while your body is restoring itself. During intense physical activity, your body's processes speed up: heart rate soars, breathing becomes heavy, and energy demands spike. After you stop exercising, your system doesn't instantly return to resting levels. Instead, you need more oxygen to:

- Replenish depleted glycogen (stored carbohydrates in muscles and liver).
- Restore normal hormone levels (adrenaline, cortisol, etc.).
- Repair muscle tissue.
- Cool the body down from elevated temperatures.

All of these tasks use energy (calories). Hence, your metabolic rate remains higher than normal for a period of time, leading to additional calorie burn.

How Significant Is the Calorie Burn?

EPOC can last anywhere from **a few hours up to 24 hours** (in some cases slightly longer).

The overall calories burned through EPOC typically represent a small but meaningful boost to your daily energy expenditure—anywhere from an extra 6% to 15% of the calories burned during the exercise session itself. While it may not double your burn, these incremental benefits can add up over time, especially if you're working out consistently.

Again we can see why people with a high performance metabolic engine seem to burn calories so easily. Their bodies have been trained to operate this way consistently over time.

Tips to Maximize Your After Burn

1. Include Intensity: Whether it's sprint intervals or heavier resistance, push your body beyond its comfort zone a few times a week.
2. Focus on Compound Movements: Exercises like squats, lunges, push-ups, and rows engage multiple muscle groups at once, requiring more energy during and after your workout.
3. Prioritize Recovery: Don't forget protein and rest! Your body needs proper nutrition and sleep to repair muscle tissue and fully recover, which can help sustain your elevated metabolic rate.
4. Stay Hydrated: Hydration supports all metabolic processes, including the post-workout recovery that fuels EPOC.

Types of Workouts That Maximize EPOC

- Heavy Resistance Training: Lifting weights with higher loads (fewer reps but more intensity) can create a significant metabolic disturbance, prolonging the after burn.
- High-Intensity Interval Training (HIIT): Alternating between short bursts of intense effort and brief rest periods spikes your heart rate multiple times, amplifying EPOC.
- Circuit Training: Moving quickly between exercises with minimal rest keeps your heart rate elevated and can extend the time your body needs to recover post-workout.

Let's take a closer look at HIIT – one of the most efficient and effective workouts for torching calories and fat.

What is HIIT (High-Intensity Interval Training)?

High-Intensity Interval Training (HIIT) is a workout method that involves short bursts of intense exercise followed by brief periods of rest or low-intensity recovery. This cycle is repeated multiple times, making HIIT one of the best ways to burn fat, build endurance, and improve cardiovascular health as well as building lean muscle.

Unlike steady-state cardio (like jogging at a moderate pace for 30 minutes), HIIT pushes your body to work at near-maximum "all-out" effort in short intervals, followed by just enough recovery time to catch your breath before the next round.

Why is HIIT So Effective?

1. Maximizes Fat Burning in Less Time: HIIT burns more calories in a shorter time than steady-state cardio. Studies show that 20-30 minutes of HIIT can burn as many calories as an hour of steady exercise.
2. Triggers the Afterburn Effect (EPOC): HIIT increases Excess Post-Exercise Oxygen Consumption (EPOC), meaning your body continues to burn calories for hours after you stop exercising. This makes HIIT a powerful metabolism booster even when you're resting.
3. Preserves Muscle While Burning Fat: Unlike excessive cardio, which can lead to muscle loss, HIIT helps maintain and even build lean muscle while shedding fat.
4. Improves Cardiovascular & Metabolic Health: HIIT strengthens your heart and lungs, improving endurance and oxygen efficiency. It boosts insulin sensitivity, helping your body process glucose more effectively (important for preventing diabetes and managing weight).
5. Time-Efficient & No Equipment Needed: HIIT workouts can be done in as little as 20-30 minutes. You don't need a gym—many HIIT exercises rely on bodyweight movements like squats, burpees, and push-ups.

How to Structure a HIIT Workout

A typical HIIT workout consists of **work intervals** (where you go all-out) and **rest intervals** (where you recover). The most common formats include:

- 30:30 (30 seconds work, 30 seconds rest) – Good for beginners.

- 40:20 (40 seconds work, 20 seconds rest) – Intermediate level.
- 45:15 or 50:10 – Advanced levels with minimal recovery.
- Tabata (20 seconds work, 10 seconds rest, repeated for 4 minutes) – One of the most intense HIIT protocols.

Example 30-Minute HIIT Routine:

ROUND 1: Lower Body (10 mins)

- Squat to Jump Squat – 40 sec work / 20 sec rest
- Reverse Lunge to Knee Drive (Right Leg) – 40 sec work / 20 sec rest
- Reverse Lunge to Knee Drive (Left Leg) – 40 sec work / 20 sec rest
- Glute Bridge March – 40 sec work / 20 sec rest
- Jumping Jacks or High Knees – 40 sec work / 20 sec rest

Rest 1 Minute

ROUND 2: Upper Body & Core (10 mins)

- Push-Ups – 40 sec work / 20 sec rest
- Plank Shoulder Taps – 40 sec work / 20 sec rest
- Superman Lifts – 40 sec work / 20 sec rest
- Bicycle Crunches – 40 sec work / 20 sec rest
- Mountain Climbers – 40 sec work / 20 sec rest

Rest 1 Minute

ROUND 3: Full Body Burn (10 mins)

- Burpees – 40 sec work / 20 sec rest

- Kettlebell Swings (or Dumbbell Swings) – 40 sec work / 20 sec rest
- Plank to Squat Jump – 40 sec work / 20 sec rest
- Russian Twists – 40 sec work / 20 sec rest
- Jump Rope or Fast Feet – 40 sec work / 20 sec rest

Cool Down & Stretch – 5 Minutes

Precautions & Who Should Avoid HIIT

If you have joint issues, heart conditions, or are new to exercise, start slowly and choose low-impact modifications. Overdoing HIIT can lead to burnout or injury. Limit sessions to 2-3 times per week, alternating with strength training and recovery days. Always warm up before and cool down after to prevent injuries.

Why 30 Minutes is Enough

A common myth is that you need to work out for an hour or more to see results. The truth? A well-structured, **EFFICIENT** 30-minute workout is more than enough to build muscle, boost metabolism, and burn fat. It's all about working smarter, not longer.

Why? Firstly, higher intensity equals greater results. A focused, high-intensity 30-minute session can be far more effective than an hour of low-effort exercise. Also, shorter workouts are easier to stick with. And you're more likely to be consistent if your workout doesn't feel like a time-consuming chore. It's not about how long you work out in a single session—it's about showing up regularly.

With the right structure, 30 minutes is all you need to see progress and grow leaner.

What about Flexibility, Mobility & Posture?

If you feel sore and stiff after high intensity training, activities like yoga can help loosen things up and keep your joints happy. Yoga brings in an element of flexibility and mobility that no other workout can quite match. It stretches and lengthens muscles, helping to release tension and stiffness while improving overall range of motion. It's also fantastic for posture—when you hold poses like downward dog or warrior, you're not just stretching, you're also strengthening key muscles that keep you upright and balanced.

Pilates is all about controlled movements that strengthen the deep stabilizing muscles, especially in the core. When your core is strong, everything else follows—your posture improves, your lower back has better support, and your balance gets better. If you've ever felt tight or weak in your lower back, or if you find yourself slouching after a long day at a desk, Pilates can be a game-changer. It teaches the body how to move with better alignment, so you're not just stronger, but also more efficient in your everyday movements.

Both Pilates and yoga teach body awareness, making you more in tune with how you move. This awareness translates into better workouts, better posture, and even better breathing. And since both are low-impact, they're gentle on the joints while still giving you a serious workout. Whether you're trying to build strength, prevent injury, or just move through life feeling more agile and pain-free, incorporating either Pilates or yoga into your routine can make a noticeable difference.

Best Workouts for Different Goals

Depending on your fitness goals, different types of workouts will serve you best. Here's how to tailor your routine:

Fitness Goal	Recommended Training	Best Exercises	Workout Frequency
Build Muscle & Boost Metabolism	Strength / Resistance training (weights, bodyweight, resistance bands)	Squats, deadlifts, push-ups, pull-ups, lunges	3-4 times per week
Lose Fat & Improve Endurance	High-Intensity Interval Training (HIIT) or Cross-fit	Kettlebell swings, burpees, sprint intervals, jump squats	2-3 times per week
Improve Flexibility & Mobility	Yoga, stretching, & mobility drills	Yoga flows, dynamic stretching, foam rolling	1-2 times per week alongside other training

Where's the Cardio?

You might be wondering why traditional cardio workouts like running, spinning, aerobics, kickboxing, or Zumba aren't at the core of this program. The simple answer? They're just not as efficient when it comes to achieving the most common fitness goals—fat loss, muscle toning, and metabolism boosting.

Let's break it down. Cardio-based exercises primarily focus on burning calories in the moment, but they don't do much to increase muscle mass or significantly boost metabolism long-term. While running for an hour may burn a substantial amount of calories, once you stop, the calorie burn stops too. Compare that to strength training or HIIT, where your body continues to burn calories for hours after your workout, thanks to the afterburn effect.

Another reason I don't prioritize these workouts is injury risk. Running, for example, is notorious for knee, hip, and joint problems, especially for women as we age. The repetitive impact of pounding the pavement can take a toll on the body, leading to shin splints, tendonitis, or even stress fractures. Spinning and aerobics classes can also be high-impact on joints, and overdoing them can lead to muscle imbalances (think: overdeveloped quads and weak hamstrings in cyclists).

That's not to say you should never do cardio. If you genuinely love running, Zumba, or kickboxing, and it brings you joy, by all means, keep doing it! Exercise should be enjoyable. But if your main goal is losing weight, sculpting your body, and improving metabolism, prioritizing strength training and HIIT or cross-fit will give you better results in less time.

Think of cardio as the cherry on top rather than the foundation. A brisk walk, a fun dance class, or an occasional run is great for overall health—but for real body transformation, muscle-building workouts should take center stage.

Tailoring Your Routine to Your Fitness Level and Schedule

The best workout plan is the one that fits your lifestyle. Here's how to customize your approach:

- Beginners: Start with 3-4 days per week of full-body strength training.
- Intermediate: Increase to 4-5 days per week, incorporating resistance training and HIIT.
- Advanced: Aim for 5-6 days per week, rotating between strength training, HIIT, and flexibility work.

Remember, it's not about perfection—it's about progress.

Train Smarter, Not Longer

The key to seeing real results isn't about spending endless hours working out—it's about choosing the most effective types of exercise that give you the biggest return on your effort. Strength training, HIIT, and mobility work like Pilates or yoga help shape your body, boost metabolism, and keep you strong and injury-free far better than traditional cardio alone.

The best workout plan is one that fits into your life sustainably. It doesn't have to be complicated or time-consuming—30 minutes of focused movement is all it takes.

Don't worry about following a "perfect" routine. Just show up, move with intention, and stay consistent. Your body will thank you —not just today, but for years to come.

Chapter 11
Timing Your Workout

When you exercise matters

Just like eating at the right time can optimize digestion and metabolism, timing your workouts correctly can enhance fat-burning and muscle-building. If you've ever tried exercising on an empty stomach and felt sluggish, now you know why! Your body needs fuel to perform optimally, and eating a well-balanced brunch before exercise makes a difference.

That's why the Brunch Yourself Thin method suggests working out after brunch (or lunch), rather than first thing in the morning on an empty stomach.

Here's a reminder of the holistic routine:

1. **A High-Protein Brunch** – A protein-packed meal kickstarts metabolism, stabilizes blood sugar, and gives you the calories you need to fuel a high intensity workout effectively.

2. **Muscle-Building Exercise** – Draws on the insulin you released and the glucose you consumed at brunch (and stored glycogen) to maximize your performance and prevent muscle breakdown. The body then utilizes amino acids from the protein to repair and strengthen muscles.
3. **A Light Lunch** – Aids the repair process to maximize muscle growth and body toning. This meal replenishes glycogen stores and provides additional protein to enhance recovery.
4. **A Balanced Dinner**
5. **An Overnight Fast**

Hopefully it's becoming clear why exercising mid-day after brunch is optimal. Because…

- Exercising after a high-protein meal ensures better performance – Your muscles are primed for movement when they have a fresh supply of amino acids from protein.
- Strength training (and muscle growth) benefits from post-meal insulin release – Insulin helps shuttle nutrients into your muscles, aiding in recovery and muscle growth.

Alternatively, if working out in the afternoons or evenings works better for your schedule – it's always better to do whatever is most sustainable. As long as your meals are packed with protein, that's the most important thing.

But Doesn't "Fasted Exercise" Burn A Lot of Fat?

Yes, exercising in a fasted state—typically in the morning before eating—can enhance fat burning, and even boost metabolic flexibility. This approach works by forcing the body to rely more on stored fat for energy rather than readily available glucose from a recent meal (as we discussed in Chapter 4).

You can certainly incorporate fasted workouts into your routine if it suits your goals; just be aware that **fasted workouts won't help you to optimally build muscle**… which is the key to maximising your metabolic engine.

The best type of exercise for fasted workouts is low- to moderate-intensity (e.g., brisk walking, cycling, steady-state jogging, yoga, or Pilates).

Avoid fasted exercise if you're doing heavy strength training (muscle repair requires amino acids from food) or other high intensity workouts like HIIT or circuit training.

How to Optimize Fasted Workouts

- Hydrate first – Drink water, black coffee, or unsweetened tea to stay energized.
- Keep it short and moderate – 20-45 minutes is usually enough.
- Break your fast with protein – Eat a protein-rich brunch after your workout to aid muscle recovery.

Chapter 12
Real Life Routines

One of the best things about Brunch Yourself Thin is that it isn't a rigid, one-size-fits-all approach. It's flexible, designed to fit seamlessly into real women's lives, regardless of their schedules or responsibilities.

Let's meet three women who follow this method in their own way.

The Work-From-Homer: A Structured, Strength-Focused Routine

Emma, 51, runs her own business from home. She loves the flexibility of setting her schedule, but she also knows how easy it is to let work creep into every part of her day. To keep herself accountable, she follows the Brunch Yourself Thin method exactly as it's designed.

She starts her day with black coffee, not really feeing hungry. By 10:30 AM, she's ready for a high-protein brunch—scrambled eggs with spinach, smoked salmon, and avocado.

At 11:30 AM, she heads to the gym for a strength training session, lifting weights to build muscle and keep her metabolism humming. She knows that muscle burns more calories at rest, so she prioritizes resistance exercises like squats, deadlifts, and rows.

Her 1:30 PM lunch is light but nourishing—grilled chicken with a big green salad, olive oil, and a handful of almonds. It's light, protein-packed, and helps her recover and repair from her workout. She spends the afternoon working, sipping tea, and feeling focused, without the mid-afternoon crash she used to get from snacking on sugary treats.

By 6:00 PM, she sits down with her family for dinner— spaghetti with lean beef and mushroom bolognese and a side salad. She enjoys her meal without stress, knowing that her overnight fast will soon begin, giving her body time to reset and metabolize efficiently.

The New Mom: Fuelling with Smart Carbs and HIIT Workouts

Sophie, 32, has a two-year-old son who keeps her on her toes all day. She loves the idea of intermittent fasting, but she also knows she needs enough energy to keep up with her little one.

Instead of a purely high-protein brunch, she adds some smart carbs to the mix. At 10:30 AM, she has some comforting porridge oats with high protein Greek yogurt and berries. This keeps her feeling satisfied but doesn't leave her sluggish.

At 12:00 PM, when her baby goes down for his nap, she gets moving and taps into those carbs with a 30-minute HIIT session in front of the TV with her favourite fitness influencer. Burpees, lunges, and push ups—she keeps it short and intense, knowing that HIIT workouts burn calories long after she's finished.

By 1:30 PM, she's ready for a quick and easy lunch—a tuna wrap with greens and hummus. It's nourishing and keeps her fuelled for the rest of the day.

Dinner at 6:00 PM is baked chicken with brown rice and roasted vegetables with a little bit of ice cream to finish—balanced but easy to prepare, so she can spend more time with her family. As her baby drifts off to sleep, Sophie enjoys a cup of herbal tea and relaxes, letting her overnight fast begin without feeling deprived.

The 9 to 5 Commuter: Making It Work in a Busy Office Life

Anna, 45, has a packed schedule. Between meetings, commuting, and picking up her kids from school, her time is limited. But she's found a way to make the Brunch Yourself Thin method work for her lifestyle.

When her scheduled is really packed, she starts her morning with fasted yoga at 6:30 AM. The gentle movement wakes her up, stretches her muscles, and helps her burn fat without needing fuel.

Instead of eating right away, she drinks green tea, waiting until 10:30 AM for brunch—a high-protein smoothie she brought with her to the office.

She keeps lunch at 1:00 PM simple and convenient—a hearty lentil soup and a few squares of dark chocolate. She avoids anything too carb-heavy, knowing she needs steady energy to power through her busy afternoon.

By 6:00 PM, she's home and ready for a balanced dinner before fasting. It's taco night and Dad's turn to cook. That calls for some skinny margaritas!

One Method, Endless Flexibility

The beauty of Brunch Yourself Thin is that it's not about rules—it's about real life. Some days are perfect for strength training, others for HIIT, while others might start with just some quick and easy mobility stretches.

Whether you're working from home, chasing toddlers, or powering through a demanding job, this method adapts to your lifestyle, making sustainable weight loss and metabolic health easier than ever.

Chapter 13
5 Habits That Change Everything

Before we move on, it's time to summarise the key points we've discussed so far, and in doing so, I'm going to ask you to make 5 promises to yourself.

More specifically, I want you to remember these 5 habits, and if you stick with them, you are guaranteed to speed up your metabolism and transform your figure. Here they are.

5 HABITS THAT CHANGE EVERYTHING

To Rest My Metabolism, I Will:

1. **Delay my first calories until a mid-morning brunch.**
2. **Get more protein into my meals.**
3. **Build muscle to burn fat.**
4. **Stop snacking, especially on sugar.**
5. **Close the kitchen after a balanced dinner.**

That's it! Can you do that? Of course you can. And if you cheat… that's okay. Just come back to the 5 habits again. In the long term, when your metabolic engine is running like a super-car… you'll notice that you can cheat quite often and it will make little difference at all. Just imagine that…!

Make A Difference With Your Review

Imagine someone just like you—scrolling through weight loss titles, unsure where to begin.

Well you can help! If you've found value in this book so far, would you take one minute to leave a review?

It costs nothing, takes almost no time, and could make a huge difference to someone's life.

Your review could be the reason someone...

☑ Finally quits binging in the evenings.

☑ Sees their waistline shrink for the first time in years.

☑ Fits into the jeans they haven't worn since college.

☑ Enjoys food again, without feeling guilty.

☑ Or adds ten healthy, vibrant years to their life!

Books like this spread because of readers like you. If you think others would benefit from the Brunch Yourself Thin method, your review helps more than you know!

Simply scan the QR Code and share your thoughts.

US Readers:
Scan for amazon.com/gp/css/order-history

UK Readers:
Scan for amazon.co.uk/gp/css/order-history

Thank you for being a part of this community! 🩶

Chapter 14
Metabolism & Menopause

What Happens to Our Metabolism in Our 40s and 50s?

If you've hit your 40s or 50s and feel like your metabolism suddenly took an extended vacation, you're not alone. Maybe you've noticed that weight creeps on more easily, especially around your belly, even though your diet and exercise haven't changed much. Or perhaps you feel like your energy levels are playing a cruel game of hide-and-seek. You're eating healthy, moving your body, and still—nothing seems to budge. Sound familiar?

That's because your metabolism is shifting, and hormones are playing a bigger role than ever before. Estrogen and progesterone levels start fluctuating, insulin sensitivity decreases, and muscle mass naturally declines if you don't actively work to maintain it. Translation? Your body is changing how it stores fat, burns energy, and regulates appetite.

Now, don't panic! This doesn't mean weight gain is inevitable or that you have to accept feeling sluggish forever. It just means your approach needs to evolve. The old tricks that worked in your 20s and 30s—cutting calories, doing more cardio—aren't necessarily the best strategies anymore. Instead, this phase of life is all about hormonal balance, smart nutrition, and muscle preservation.

The good news? You're not powerless. By following the Brunch Yourself Thin routine, you can support your metabolism, feel stronger, and even reverse some of the common struggles of menopause.

1. A 16-Hour Fast Supports Hormonal Balance

Intermittent fasting isn't just about weight loss—it's a powerful tool for balancing hormones and improving metabolic health, especially during menopause. A 16-hour fast followed by an 8-hour eating window can help regulate hormones that influence weight, appetite, and energy levels.

- Improves Insulin Sensitivity – Declining estrogen can make the body more prone to insulin resistance, leading to fat storage around the belly. A 16-hour fast gives insulin levels time to drop, making the body more efficient at burning fat.
- Reduces Inflammation – Chronic inflammation is linked to many menopausal symptoms, including weight gain and fatigue. Fasting triggers cellular repair and lowers inflammation.
- Balances Cortisol – Fasting can help stabilize cortisol levels, preventing stress-related weight gain. However, it's important to avoid extreme fasting, which could increase cortisol instead of balancing it.

- Boosts Growth Hormone – Growth hormone declines with age, but fasting naturally boosts its production, supporting muscle maintenance and fat loss.
- Supports Gut Health – The fasting period allows the gut to rest and reset, improving digestion and nutrient absorption.

The key to making a 16-hour fast work for you is listening to your body. The goal is to use fasting as a tool for hormone regulation, not as a form of restriction.

2. Prioritize Protein to Preserve Muscle Mass

Eating enough protein is one of the most effective ways to fight age-related muscle loss and maintain a strong metabolism. Aim for 25-30 grams of protein per meal to keep muscles strong and support fat burning.

Best protein sources:

- Lean meats (chicken, turkey, grass-fed beef)
- Fatty fish (salmon, sardines, tuna)
- Eggs
- Greek yogurt & cottage cheese
- Tofu, tempeh & legumes
- Protein shakes (when needed for convenience)

3. Strength Training is Non-Negotiable

Since we naturally lose muscle as we age, strength training is essential. Lifting weights 2-4 times per week can help maintain muscle tone, bone density, and a faster metabolism. Focus on compound exercises like squats, lunges, deadlifts, and push-ups to target multiple muscle groups efficiently.

4. Control Blood Sugar with Smart Carbs

Women in their 40s and 50s become more sensitive to carbs, so eating the right kind of carbohydrates is key. Instead of highly processed foods, opt for:

- Whole grains (quinoa, brown rice, oats)
- Non-starchy vegetables (leafy greens, peppers, zucchini)
- Legumes & beans (black beans, chickpeas, lentils)
- Berries (blueberries, raspberries, strawberries)

Pairing carbs with protein and fiber helps prevent blood sugar spikes and cravings.

5. Manage Stress & Cortisol Levels

Higher stress hormones (cortisol) during menopause can increase belly fat and disrupt sleep. Managing stress is just as important as diet and exercise for weight management. Helpful strategies include:

- Mindful movement (yoga, Pilates, or stretching)
- Meditation & deep breathing exercises
- Prioritizing quality sleep (7-9 hours per night)
- Walking outdoors (daily sunlight exposure regulates hormones)

6. Supplement Smartly

While whole foods should always be the foundation of good nutrition, some key supplements can support metabolism and hormone balance during this stage of life.

Best Supplements for Menopause & Metabolism:

- Magnesium – Supports muscle function, reduces stress, and improves sleep.
- Vitamin D3 + K2 – Essential for bone health and immune function.
- Omega-3s (Fish Oil) – Helps fight inflammation and supports heart health.
- Collagen – Supports skin, joints, and muscle repair.
- B Vitamins – Helps energy production and metabolism.
- Probiotics – Supports gut health and digestion, which can become sluggish with age.

Thriving Through Menopause

Menopause doesn't mean you have to accept weight gain, fatigue, or a sluggish metabolism. By making these smart adjustments to your diet, exercise routine, and stress management habits, you can support your metabolism and feel your best in your 40s, 50s, and beyond.

The key is to focus on muscle maintenance, hormonal balance, and blood sugar control while embracing a lifestyle that feels sustainable and enjoyable. Aging is inevitable, but struggling with weight and energy doesn't have to be. With the strategies in this book, you can stay strong, lean, and vibrant for decades to come.

Chapter 15
Mindset & Motivation

Going Off Track

It happens to everyone. You're following the plan, seeing progress, and then—boom! Life gets in the way. A stressful week at work, a vacation filled with indulgence, or just a phase where motivation disappears. Going off track is part of the process, and the key to long-term success isn't perfection—it's learning how to reset and keep moving forward.

Common Triggers That Can Derail Progress

- Emotional Eating: Stress, boredom, or sadness can make you reach for food as comfort rather than nourishment.
- Unrealistic Expectations: If you expect rapid results, it's easy to feel discouraged when progress slows.
- Over-Restricting Food Choices: Cutting out all your favorite foods often backfires, leading to binge-eating or cravings.

- Lack of Routine: Skipping meals, inconsistent fasting windows, or missing workouts can throw your body off balance.
- Social Pressures: Dining out, special events, and well-meaning friends offering tempting foods can challenge your willpower.

The solution? Anticipate these triggers and have a plan to navigate them instead of letting them undo your progress.

Overcoming Emotional Eating & Stress

Food is deeply connected to emotions, and sometimes we eat not because we're hungry, but because we're stressed, bored, or overwhelmed. Instead of turning to food as a comfort, try these alternatives:

- Identify Triggers: Keep a journal to track when and why emotional eating happens.
- Find Non-Food Rewards: A bath, a walk, a good book, or even a phone call to a friend can provide comfort without food.
- Use Mindful Eating Techniques: Before eating, ask yourself: "Am I truly hungry, or am I just seeking comfort?"
- Keep Healthier Comfort Foods On Hand: If you need something, have protein-rich snacks like Greek yogurt, almonds, or dark chocolate available instead of processed treats.
- Practice Stress Reduction Daily: Yoga, meditation, deep breathing, or simply taking 10 minutes to relax can prevent stress from triggering overeating.

Breaking Plateaus: What To Do When Progress Stalls

At some point, the scale may stop moving, and fat loss might slow down. This doesn't mean what you're doing isn't working—it just means your body has adapted, and it's time to make a few strategic changes.

Extending Your Fasting Window

Think of your metabolism like a thermostat. When it gets too comfortable at a certain setting, it stops working as hard. But if you make a slight adjustment—just enough to shake things up—you encourage your body to burn through stored fat again. Extending your fast is one of the simplest ways to do this.

You've already been fasting for 16 hours with the Brunch Yourself Thin method. By stretching it just a little longer—to 18 or even 20 hours—you can push your body deeper into fat-burning mode without drastically changing what you eat.

Why Does This Work? When you extend your fast, your body burns through more of its glycogen stores, forcing it to tap into fat for energy. It also increases autophagy, which helps clean out damaged cells and improve metabolism. It enhances insulin sensitivity, making it easier for your body to use food efficiently once you eat again. And it further boosts human growth hormone (HGH), which supports muscle retention and fat loss.The key is that this isn't starvation—it's just giving your body a little extra time to reset before you eat again.

If you're used to breaking your fast at 10:30 AM, try pushing back a few hours for a few days per week. That's an 18-hour fast instead of 16. If you feel good and want to go further, try extending to 2:30 PM for a 20 hour fast.

Here's a simple schedule:

Option 1: 18-Hour Fast

- First Meal (12:30 PM): A high-protein, balanced lunch
- Workout (1:00 PM): Strength training or HIIT
- Snack (3:30 PM): Something light & protein-rich
- Second Meal (6:00 PM): A balanced family dinner
- Fast from 6:30 PM to 12:30 PM (18 hours)

Option 2: 20-Hour Fast (for more advanced fasting)

- First Meal (2:30 PM): A nutrient-dense lunch with healthy fats (e.g., eggs, avocado, smoked salmon)
- Workout (4:00 PM): Strength training or a brisk walk
- Second Meal (6:00 PM): A balanced family dinner before fasting begins again
- Fast from 6:30 PM to 2:30 PM (20 hours)

This isn't something you have to do every day, but even two to three days per week can help break through a plateau without requiring a major diet overhaul.

A Note on Longer Fasts

While intermittent fasting can be a powerful tool for weight management, metabolic health, and longevity, prolonged fasting (beyond 16–24 hours) may not be suitable for everyone. The long-term effects of extended fasting are still being studied, and individual responses can vary based on factors like age, medical history, and activity level.

If you have any underlying health conditions, are pregnant, breast-feeding, or taking medication, it's always best to consult with your healthcare professional before making significant changes to your eating patterns. Fasting should support your health, not compromise it—so listen to your body, and approach any adjustments with care.

Reassess Your Macros

- Increase Protein Intake: Protein supports muscle maintenance and fat loss. If you've plateaued, increasing your protein by 5-10g per meal could help.
- Be Mindful of Hidden Carbs & Sugars: Even "healthy" foods like fruit smoothies or energy bars can slow progress if consumed too often.

Change Up Your Workout Routine

- Incorporate More Strength Training: If you've been doing mostly cardio, adding resistance training can help build muscle and speed up metabolism.
- Increase Workout Intensity: Try heavier weights, shorter rest periods, or a mix of HIIT and strength training to challenge your body in new ways.
- Add Movement Throughout the Day: Daily activity beyond your workouts—like walking, stretching, or standing more—can make a difference.

Track Trends, Not Just the Scale

- Look at Non-Scale Victories: Are your clothes fitting better? Are you feeling stronger and more energized?

- Take Progress Photos & Measurements: Sometimes fat loss is happening, but the scale isn't showing it.
- Monitor Your Energy Levels & Sleep: If you're always tired, it might mean your body needs more recovery rather than further calorie cutting.

Setting Sustainable Goals

Fat loss is not a straight path. There will be ups, downs, fast progress, and slow periods. What keeps people successful is having realistic and sustainable goals.

1. Shift From Outcome Goals to Habit Goals

- Instead of saying, "I want to lose 10 pounds," say, "I will strength train 3 times per week."
- Instead of focusing on, "I need to fit into a size 6," focus on, "I will eat 30g of protein per meal."

2. Celebrate Small Wins

- Did you stick to your fasting window all week? That's a win.
- Did you meal prep instead of ordering takeout? Another win.
- Did you lift heavier weights or complete a workout you couldn't do before? Huge win.

3. Accept That Perfection Isn't the Goal

- Long-term success is about consistency, not being perfect.
- One missed workout or one indulgent meal doesn't undo progress—what you do most of the time matters more.

Keep Moving Forward

Everyone hits setbacks, plateaus, and moments of frustration. What separates those who succeed from those who give up is the ability to adjust and keep going. Your body is always changing, adapting, and responding to your habits. If something stops working, tweak it. If you go off track, reset.

This journey isn't about dieting forever—it's about creating a lifestyle that keeps you feeling strong, lean, and confident for years to come.

Chapter 16
The Habit Challenge

Why Journaling Your 3Ps Brunch Can Help Build a Lasting Habit

One of the biggest challenges with any new routine is sticking with it long enough for it to become second nature. That's why tracking what you eat—not in a restrictive, obsessive way, but as a tool for awareness—can be incredibly powerful.

By journaling your 3Ps brunch (Protein, Produce, and Portion control) every day, you create a habit of mindful eating and hold yourself accountable. It's easy to assume we're eating well, but when we actually write it down, we notice patterns we might not have been aware of.

A habit isn't formed overnight. It takes repetition, consistency, and small daily wins. That's why this challenge is about more than just tracking food—it's about developing a sustainable, balanced approach to eating that aligns with your long-term goals.

Your 30-Day Brunch Challenge

This challenge is designed to help you stay consistent, accountable, and aware of your eating habits—without overcomplicating the process.

The Rules:

1. Every day for 30 days, take a photo of your brunch (or your first calories…)
2. Include a timestamp to reinforce consistency.
3. Save all your photos in a dedicated album on your phone.
4. At the end of the 30 days, reflect: What patterns do you notice? Were you eating at consistent times? Were your meals balanced? Did you feel better on certain days than others?

Why This Works

Firstly, it creates visual accountability. Seeing all your meals lined up over the course of a month shows your progress in a way numbers on a scale never could.

It also builds awareness. You'll quickly notice trends—are you really getting enough protein? Are you reaching for sugar more often than you thought?

And it motivates consistency. When you've built up a streak of 10, 15, or 20 days, you won't want to break it.

This isn't about perfection—it's about progress. If you miss a day, don't quit. Just keep going.

By the end of the 30 days, you'll have built a sustainable habit of planning balanced meals, being mindful of your food choices, and staying consistent—without stress or deprivation.

Are you ready to take the challenge?

Chapter 17
A New Blueprint for Modern Women

Throughout this book, we've explored a sustainable, realistic, and science-backed approach to optimizing metabolism, balancing hormones, and maintaining a healthy weight without restrictive dieting.

The Brunch Yourself Thin protocol is more than just an eating schedule—it's a shift in mindset. By prioritizing a high-protein brunch, efficient strength training, smart carb choices, and a structured fasting window, you give your body the fuel it needs while tapping into its natural fat-burning capabilities.

The Key Benefits of the Brunch Yourself Thin Protocol are:

- Fat Loss Without Starvation: You harness the power of intermittent fasting and proper meal timing to encourage fat loss without feeling deprived.
- Optimized Hormones & Metabolism: Fasting, strength training, and nutrient-dense meals help regulate insulin,

cortisol, and hunger hormones to support long-term weight management.
- Increased Energy & Mental Clarity: By reducing blood sugar spikes and focusing on whole, unprocessed foods, you avoid energy crashes and improve focus throughout the day.
- A Flexible, Family-Friendly Approach: Unlike traditional diet plans, this method allows you to enjoy dinner with your family while still achieving metabolic balance.
- Sustainable & Adaptable: Whether you work from home, juggle a 9-to-5, or have young kids, the principles of this plan can be tailored to fit your life.

Reclaiming Health & Vitality at Any Age

This book isn't just about losing weight—it's about reclaiming control over how you feel, move, and fuel your body at every stage of life. Your metabolism, energy levels, and strength don't have to decline with age. With simple yet effective strategies, you can maintain muscle, manage hormones, and build a healthier future.

Next Steps: Putting This Blueprint Into Action

It's time to commit to the Brunch Yourself Thin Method. Implement the 5 habits recommended in this book and don't worry if you go off track every now and then.

Track your progress by using the habit challenge or journal your meals to build awareness and accountability. Stay flexible and consistent. Remember, perfection isn't the goal and you can adapt the plan to fit your lifestyle.

As you go, listen to your body. Adjust your fasting window, meal choices, and workouts based on how you feel. And don't forget to celebrate your wins! Progress isn't only measured by the scale or the measuring tape. Focus on other victories like better energy, improved digestion, and greater strength as well.

You now have a blueprint for resetting your metabolic engine to super-car mode, the key to achieving the figure you've always wanted. Whether you're just getting started or fine-tuning your routine, this journey is about finding what works for you and making it a lifelong habit.

Your health is in your hands—so go forward with confidence, stay consistent, and enjoy the transformation ahead!

Appendices

Appendix 1: A Sample 7-Day Meal Plan

This 7-day meal plan is designed to fit within the Brunch Yourself Thin framework, incorporating high-protein brunches, light lunches, and family-friendly dinners, all while following the 16:8 intermittent fasting schedule.

Day 1

Brunch (10:30 AM): Scrambled eggs with smoked salmon, avocado, and sautéed spinach.

- *Prep time:* 5 minutes | *Cook time:* 5 minutes
- *Recipe:* Heat a pan over medium heat, melt 1 tsp butter, and scramble 2 eggs. Add smoked salmon in the last 30 seconds of cooking. Serve with half an avocado and sautéed spinach cooked in olive oil for 2-3 minutes.

Lunch (1:30 PM): Grilled chicken salad with mixed greens, walnuts, feta, and balsamic dressing.

- *Prep time:* 10 minutes | *Cook time:* 10 minutes
- *Recipe:* Grill a chicken breast over medium-high heat for 5 minutes per side until fully cooked. Slice and toss with mixed greens, 1 tbsp walnuts, and 1 tbsp crumbled feta. Drizzle with balsamic dressing.

Dinner (6:00 PM): Spaghetti Bolognese with a side salad.

- *Prep time:* 10 minutes | *Cook time:* 30 minutes
- *Recipe:* In a pan, cook 1 lb lean ground beef with 1 chopped onion and 2 minced garlic cloves over medium heat until browned. Add 1 can diced tomatoes, 1 cup tomato sauce, 1 tsp oregano, and ½ tsp salt. Simmer for 20 minutes. Serve over whole wheat or lentil pasta with a side salad.

Day 2

Brunch: Greek yogurt with almonds, chia seeds, and mixed berries.

- *Prep time:* 2 minutes | *Cook time:* None
- *Recipe:* Mix 1 cup Greek yogurt with 1 tbsp chia seeds, 1 tbsp almonds, and a handful of mixed berries.

Lunch: Turkey and avocado lettuce wraps with a side of cucumber and hummus.

- *Prep time:* 5 minutes | *Cook time:* None
- *Recipe:* Wrap sliced turkey and avocado in large lettuce leaves. Serve with sliced cucumber and 2 tbsp hummus.

Dinner: Roast chicken with mashed potatoes and steamed vegetables.

- *Prep time:* 10 minutes | *Cook time:* 60 minutes | *Oven temperature:* 375°F (190°C)
- *Recipe:* Rub a whole chicken with olive oil, salt, pepper, and garlic. Roast for 1 hour or until internal temperature reaches 165°F (75°C). Serve with mashed potatoes (boiled and mashed with butter) and steamed carrots and broccoli.

Day 3

Brunch: Omelet with mushrooms, tomatoes, and goat cheese.

- *Prep time:* 5 minutes | *Cook time:* 5 minutes
- *Recipe:* Whisk 2 eggs and cook in a pan over medium heat. Add sautéed mushrooms, tomatoes, and 1 tbsp goat cheese before folding.

Lunch: Quinoa bowl with black beans, cherry tomatoes, and grilled shrimp.

- *Prep time:* 10 minutes | *Cook time:* 15 minutes
- *Recipe:* Cook ½ cup quinoa according to package instructions. Toss with black beans, cherry tomatoes, and grilled shrimp seasoned with lime juice.

Dinner: Cottage Pie with a side of carrots.

- *Prep time:* 15 minutes | *Cook time:* 30 minutes | *Oven temperature:* 375°F (190°C)
- *Recipe:* Brown 1 lb ground turkey or beef with onions and garlic. Add 1 cup peas and carrots, then place in a baking dish. Top with mashed potatoes and bake for 20 minutes.

Day 4

Brunch: Chia pudding with coconut milk, topped with walnuts and fresh fruit.

- *Prep time:* 5 minutes | *Rest time:* 4 hours (or overnight)
- *Recipe:* Mix 3 tbsp chia seeds with 1 cup coconut milk. Let sit overnight. Top with walnuts and fresh fruit.

Lunch: Tuna salad with mixed greens and olive oil dressing.

- *Prep time:* 5 minutes | *Cook time:* None
- *Recipe:* Mix 1 can tuna with 1 tbsp olive oil. Serve over mixed greens.

Dinner: Homemade Tacos with Ground Beef and Fresh Salsa.

- *Prep time:* 10 minutes | *Cook time:* 20 minutes
- *Recipe:* Cook 1 lb ground beef with taco seasoning. Serve in corn tortillas with shredded lettuce, diced tomatoes, and fresh salsa.

Day 5

Brunch: Protein smoothie (almond milk, protein powder, peanut butter, banana, flaxseeds).

- *Prep time:* 5 minutes | *Cook time:* None
- *Recipe:* Blend 1 cup almond milk, 1 scoop protein powder, 1 tbsp peanut butter, 1 banana, and 1 tbsp flaxseeds.

Lunch: Egg salad with leafy greens and a handful of almonds.

- *Prep time:* 5 minutes | *Cook time:* 10 minutes
- *Recipe:* Mix 2 boiled eggs with Greek yogurt or mayo. Serve over leafy greens with almonds.

Dinner: Baked Salmon with Rice and Roasted Vegetables.

- *Prep time:* 10 minutes | *Cook time:* 25 minutes | *Oven temperature:* 400°F (200°C)
- *Recipe:* Bake salmon fillets with lemon and dill at 400°F (200°C) for 15-20 minutes. Serve with brown rice and roasted asparagus and carrots.

Day 6

Brunch: Cottage cheese with walnuts, cinnamon, and apple slices.

- *Prep time:* 5 minutes | *Cook time:* None
- *Recipe:* Mix 1 cup cottage cheese with 1 tbsp walnuts and a sprinkle of cinnamon. Serve with apple slices.

Dinner: Chicken Stir-Fry with Brown Rice.

- *Prep time:* 10 minutes | *Cook time:* 20 minutes
- *Recipe:* Stir-fry sliced chicken breast with bell peppers and snap peas. Serve with brown rice.

Day 7

Brunch: Scrambled tofu with mushrooms, bell peppers, and avocado.

- *Prep time:* 5 minutes | *Cook time:* 5 minutes

- *Recipe:* Sauté crumbled tofu with mushrooms, bell peppers, and seasoning. Serve with avocado.

Dinner: Family-Style Roast Beef with Sweet Potatoes.

- *Prep time:* 15 minutes | *Cook time:* 60 minutes | *Oven temperature:* 375°F (190°C)
- *Recipe:* Roast a beef joint with garlic and rosemary at 375°F (190°C) for 1 hour. Serve with mashed sweet potatoes and steamed green beans.

Homemade Smoothie Recipes

Smoothies are a great way to pack in protein, fiber, and healthy fats to keep you full and energized. Here are a few delicious and nutritious smoothie recipes to try:

1. Green Protein Power Smoothie

Prep time: 5 minutes | Servings: 1

- 1 scoop vanilla protein powder
- 1 cup unsweetened almond milk
- ½ banana
- 1 cup spinach
- ½ avocado
- 1 tbsp chia seeds
- 1 tsp honey (optional)
- 5-6 ice cubes
- Blend until smooth and enjoy!

2. Berry Antioxidant Smoothie

Prep time: 5 minutes | Servings: 1

- 1 scoop vanilla or berry-flavored protein powder
- 1 cup unsweetened coconut milk
- ½ cup frozen mixed berries
- ½ cup Greek yogurt
- 1 tbsp flaxseeds
- 5-6 ice cubes
- Blend until smooth and enjoy!

3. Peanut Butter Banana Recovery Smoothie

Prep time: 5 minutes | Servings: 1

- 1 scoop chocolate or vanilla protein powder
- 1 cup unsweetened oat milk
- 1 tbsp natural peanut butter
- 1 banana
- ½ tsp cinnamon
- 1 tbsp ground flaxseeds
- Blend until creamy and enjoy!

4. Tropical Energy Smoothie

Prep time: 5 minutes | Servings: 1

- 1 scoop vanilla protein powder
- 1 cup unsweetened coconut water
- ½ cup frozen mango
- ½ cup frozen pineapple

- 1 tbsp shredded coconut
- 1 tbsp chia seeds
- Blend and enjoy for a refreshing tropical boost!

5. Chocolate Almond Smoothie

Prep time: 5 minutes | Servings: 1

- 1 scoop chocolate protein powder
- 1 cup unsweetened almond milk
- 1 tbsp almond butter
- 1 tbsp unsweetened cocoa powder
- ½ banana
- 1 tsp honey (optional)
- Blend and enjoy a chocolatey, protein-rich treat!

These smoothies are quick, nutritious, and packed with metabolism-friendly ingredients making them an ideal way to start your day with brunch.

Meal Plan Notes:

- Hydration: Drink plenty of water throughout the day, and include herbal tea or black coffee as desired.
- Snacks (if needed): Hard-boiled eggs, a handful of nuts, or sliced veggies with hummus.
- Customization: Adjust portion sizes based on your activity level and individual needs.

This plan provides a variety of proteins, fiber-rich vegetables, and healthy fats to keep your metabolism running efficiently while keeping meals simple and delicious. Stick to this structure and adjust as needed to fit your lifestyle!

Appendix 2: Macros Reference Table

Category	Food	Protein (g)	Carbohydrates (g)	Fibre (g)	Sugar (g)	Fat (g)	Saturated Fat (g)	Glycemic Index	Glycemic Load
Proteins	Chicken Breast	31	0	0	0	3.5	1	-	-
Proteins	Salmon	25	0	0	0	13	3	-	-
Proteins	Eggs	13	1	0	1	9	3.3	-	-
Proteins	Tofu	8	2	2	0	4	0.5	-	-
Proteins	Greek Yogurt	10	4	0	4	5	3	-	-
Proteins	Ground Beef (90% lean)	24	0	0	0	10	4.5	-	-
Proteins	Turkey Breast	29	0	0	0	2	0.7	-	-
Proteins	Tuna	30	0	0	0	1	0.2	-	-
Proteins	Shrimp	24	1	0	0	1	0.3	-	-
Proteins	Lamb	25	0	0	0	16	7	-	-
Proteins	Steak	27	0	0	0	15	6	-	-
Legumes	Lentils	9	20	8	1	0.5	0.1	32	5
Legumes	Black Beans	8.9	22	7.5	1	0.7	0.2	30	6
Legumes	Chickpeas	8	27	7	2	2	0.3	28	9
Legumes	Edamame	11	9	5	2	0.2	0.1	18	3
Legumes	Peas	5	15	6	5	0.5	0.2	22	4
Legumes	Kidney Beans	7	21	8	3	0.3	0.1	29	6
Legumes	Pinto Beans	7	22	7	1	0.4	0.2	31	7
Legumes	Soybeans	16	10	8	2	0.5	0.2	20	3
Legumes	Mung Beans	14	12	9	3	0.2	0.1	23	4
Legumes	Green Beans	2	7	4	1	0.1	0	25	5
Produce	Apple	0.5	25	4.4	19	0.3	-	36	6
Produce	Banana	1.3	27	3.1	14	0.5	-	51	13
Produce	Blueberries	0.7	14	2.4	10	0.2	-	40	4
Produce	Oranges	1.2	15	3	9	0.4	-	43	7
Produce	Strawberries	0.8	9	2.1	15	0.2	-	40	5
Produce	Tomatoes	0.9	5	1.5	8	0.1	-	22	5
Produce	Carrots	0.9	10	3.6	5	0.1	-	47	3
Produce	Broccoli	2.8	7	2.6	2	0.1	-	15	2
Produce	Spinach	2.9	3	2.2	2	0.2	-	9	1
Carbohydrates	White Rice (1 cup)	2.7	45	0.6	0	0.4	0.1	73	22
Carbohydrates	Brown Rice (1 cup)	2.6	43	2.5	0	0.3	0.1	55	16
Carbohydrates	Quinoa (1 cup)	4.1	39	5.2	1	1	0.2	53	13
Carbohydrates	Instant Oats (1/4 cup dry)	2.5	27	4	0.5	1.2	0.3	83	12
Carbohydrates	Steel-Cut Oats (1/4 cup dry)	3	26	5	0.5	1.2	0.3	55	7
Carbohydrates	Whole Wheat Bread (1 slice)	8	41	3.9	2	1	0.2	74	15
Carbohydrates	Whole Wheat Pasta (1 cup)	7.5	38	4.5	0	0.5	0.1	48	18
Carbohydrates	White Pasta (1 cup cooked)	7	44	2	0	0.5	0.1	64	25
Carbohydrates	Corn Tortilla (1 medium)	6.8	30	3.1	2	1.2	0.3	52	12
Carbohydrates	Sweet Potato (1 medium)	3.4	24	3.6	1	0.2	0.1	63	14
Carbohydrates	Couscous (1 cup cooked)	5.1	29	3.8	3	0.3	0.1	65	16
Carbohydrates	Barley (1 cup cooked)	5.2	37	4.2	1	0.4	0.2	50	13
Carbohydrates	Potatoes, Boiled (1 medium)	3	37	3.8	2	0.1	0.1	58	13
Carbohydrates	French Fries (medium serving)	3	42	3.5	0	12	1.5	70	22
Dairy	Whole Milk	8	12	0	12	8	4.6	40	5
Dairy	Skim Milk	8	9	0	9	5	3.1	37	4
Dairy	Greek Yogurt (unsweetened)	10	4	0	4	5	3	11	1
Dairy	Cottage Cheese	12	3	0	3	4	2.6	10	1

Category	Item								
Dairy	Ricotta Cheese	11	4	0	4	13	8	0	0
Dairy	Cheddar Cheese	25	1	0	1	33	21	0	0
Dairy	Mozzarella Cheese	22	3	0	3	28	16	0	0
Dairy	Butter	0.9	0	0	0	81	51	0	0
Dairy	Cream Cheese	4	2	0	2	35	20	0	0
Dairy	Sour Cream	3	3	0	3	20	10	0	0
Dairy	Heavy Cream	5	2	0	2	82	51	0	0
Sugary Treats	Milk Chocolate (50g bar)	7	52	3	24	30	18	49	22
Sugary Treats	Dark Chocolate (85%) (50g)	5.4	30	5	12	25	14	23	10
Sugary Treats	Ice Cream (1 cup)	3	25	0.5	21	11	7	60	15
Sugary Treats	Candy Bar (50g)	3	60	1	24	15	9	70	30
Sugary Treats	Sugary Cereal (1 cup)	2	75	0.8	65	2	1	75	42
Sugary Treats	Donut (1 medium)	4	45	1	32	22	12	76	38
Sugary Treats	Cake (1 slice)	5	55	2	45	17	10	65	28
Sugary Treats	Cookies (2 medium)	4	48	1.5	40	14	8	69	31
Sugary Treats	Pastry (1 piece)	3.5	50	1.2	48	12	7	59	24
Sugary Treats	Milkshake (16 oz)	6	64	1.8	60	18	11	85	50

Appendix 3: FAQs About Intermittent Fasting, Meal Timing, and Hormone Health

1. What if I feel hungry in the morning?

Feeling hungry at the start of intermittent fasting is normal, especially if you're used to eating early. Your body will adapt over time. Try drinking water, black coffee, or herbal tea to help suppress hunger. Most people find that after a few days, their appetite naturally adjusts.

2. Can I drink coffee or tea while fasting?

Yes! Black coffee, unsweetened tea, and herbal tea are all fine during the fasting window. Just avoid cream, milk, sugar, or anything that contains calories, as this would break the fast.

3. What happens if I break my fast early?

It's okay! One meal or one day won't ruin your progress. Just get back on track at your next fasting window. The key is consistency over time, not perfection.

4. Will fasting slow my metabolism?

No, intermittent fasting can actually boost metabolism by increasing insulin sensitivity and promoting fat oxidation. However, chronic undereating or excessive fasting can cause the body to adapt and slow energy expenditure. A 16:8 fast strikes a balance between fasting benefits and fueling your metabolism.

5. Can I work out while fasting?

Yes, many people find that fasted workouts help burn fat more efficiently. Low to moderate intensity works best. But, if you're doing strength training, you may want to eat after your workout to aid muscle recovery. If you feel weak or fatigued, adjust your schedule to eat before training.

6. How do I prevent muscle loss while fasting?

Ensure you're eating enough protein during your eating window and incorporating strength training into your routine. Muscle loss happens primarily when fasting is combined with a low-protein, low-calorie diet.

7. Will intermittent fasting help with hormone balance?

Yes, intermittent fasting can support hormone regulation by improving insulin sensitivity, reducing inflammation, and promoting balanced cortisol levels. However, fasting should be tailored to your body's needs—overly long fasts can increase stress hormones in some women, so listening to your body is key.

8. Can intermittent fasting help during perimenopause and menopause?

Yes! Fasting can help regulate insulin, reduce belly fat, and improve energy levels—all important factors during hormonal transitions. However, if fasting leads to fatigue or worsens symptoms, adjusting the fasting window or adding more protein and healthy fats may help.

9. How do I adjust fasting if I have an irregular schedule?

Intermittent fasting is flexible! If your schedule varies, choose an eating window that fits your lifestyle. The key is to keep fasting windows consistent most days while allowing occasional adjustments.

10. Can I fast if I have thyroid issues?

If you have a thyroid condition, intermittent fasting should be approached cautiously. Some people with hypothyroidism benefit from fasting, while others may feel more fatigued. It's always best to consult your doctor and prioritize nutrient-dense meals to support thyroid function.

11. Why am I seeing changes in my poop?

Intermittent fasting and dietary changes can impact digestion. You may experience shifts in bowel movements due to:

- Increased fiber intake from more whole foods, fruits, and vegetables. Some people experience looser or more urgent bowel movements when they increase fiber intake, especially if they consume a lot of soluble fiber. And if you increase fiber intake too quickly, your digestive system may struggle to process the additional roughage, leading to bloating, gas, and mild cramping. This is because fiber feeds gut bacteria, which produce gas as a byproduct. This effect usually subsides once the gut adjusts.
- Changes in gut bacteria as your microbiome adapts to new eating patterns.
- Dehydration—make sure you're drinking enough water, especially during fasting hours.
- Lower food volume—if you're eating fewer meals, you may have less frequent bowel movements, which is normal.
- Fat adaptation—as your body burns more fat for fuel, stool consistency may change temporarily. If you experience persistent discomfort, bloating, or irregular digestion, consider adjusting your fiber intake, hydration, or meal timing.

12. How long should I fast to see results?

Most people start noticing changes in energy, digestion, and weight within 2-4 weeks. Long-term benefits like improved hormone balance and fat loss continue to build over several months.

This FAQ is meant to provide clarity, but always listen to your body and adjust your fasting approach based on what feels best for you.

Bibliography

Anton, S. D., Moehl, K., Donahoo, W. T., Marosi, K., Lee, S. A., Mainous, A. G., & Mattson, M. P. (2018). Flipping the metabolic switch: Understanding and applying the health benefits of fasting. Obesity, 26(2), 254-268. https://doi.org/10.1002/oby.22065

Astrup, A., & Raben, A. (2019). Meal timing and composition in relation to metabolic regulation and weight control. Journal of Nutrition, 149(4), 605-611. https://doi.org/10.1093/jn/nxy272

Bray, G. A., & Popkin, B. M. (2014). Dietary sugar and body weight: Have we reached a crisis in obesity? Health Affairs, 33(10), 1742-1748. https://doi.org/10.1377/hlthaff.2014.0387

Mattson, M. P., Longo, V. D., & Harvie, M. (2017). Impact of intermittent fasting on health and disease processes. Ageing Research Reviews, 39, 46-58. https://doi.org/10.1016/j.arr.2016.10.005

Johnstone, A. M. (2015). Fasting for weight loss: An effective strategy or latest dieting trend? Obesity Reviews, 16(3), 225-236. https://doi.org/10.1111/obr.12250

Slavin, J. L. (2005). Dietary fiber and body weight. Nutrition, 21(3), 411-418. https://doi.org/10.1016/j.nut.2004.08.018

Ludwig, D. S. (2002). The glycemic index: Physiological mechanisms relating to obesity, diabetes, and cardiovascular disease. Journal of the American Medical Association, 287(18), 2414-2423. https://doi.org/10.1001/jama.287.18.2414

Samaha, F. F., Iqbal, N., Seshadri, P., Chicano, K. L., Daily, D. A., McGrory, J., & Foster, G. D. (2003). A low-carbohydrate as compared with a low-fat diet in severe obesity. New England Journal of Medicine, 348(21), 2074-2081. https://doi.org/10.1056/NEJMoa022637

Hall, K. D., Bemis, T., Brychta, R., Chen, K. Y., Courville, A., & Chung, S. T. (2021). Calorie for calorie, dietary fat restriction results in more body fat loss than carbohydrate restriction in people with obesity. Cell Metabolism, 33(5), 902-914. https://doi.org/10.1016/j.cmet.2021.03.019

Roberts, S. B., & Rosenberg, I. (2006). Nutrition and aging: Changes in the regulation of energy metabolism with aging. Physiological Reviews, 86(2), 651-667. https://doi.org/10.1152/physrev.00019.2005

Printed in Great Britain
by Amazon